Empathic Communities

Empathic Communities
Educating for Justice

JOHANNA M. SELLES

With a Foreword by Margaret A. Farley

WIPF & STOCK · Eugene, Oregon

EMPATHIC COMMUNITIES
Educating for Justice

Wipf & Stock
An Imprint of Wipf and Stock Publishers
199 W. 8th Ave., Suite 3
Eugene, OR 97401

www. wipfandstock.com

ISBN 13: 978-1-60899-861-6

Manufactured in the U.S.A.

To Joan Wyatt, Emmanuel College,
in honor of her professional career
as a nurse, minister, professor,
and supporter of the arts

and to my sisters

Growth toward openness means dialogue, trusting in others, listening to them, particularly to those who say things we don't like to hear, speaking together about our mutual needs and how we might grow to new things. The birth of a good society comes when people start to trust each other, to share with each other, and to feel concerned for each other.

Jean Vanier, *Becoming Human*, 34

Contents

Foreword

EMPATHY IS A CONCEPT both revered and contested as a significant moral element in our responses to one another. Like its analogues compassion, pity, and sympathy, it is revered as a relational virtue, an illuminator of the genuine needs of others, and a motivational impetus to morally good and useful action. But also like its analogues or cognate notions, empathy is frequently disparaged as a danger to disciplined caring, especially in contexts where professional expertise requires emotional discipline, clear-sighted focus, and absolute attention to a task at hand. Fear of empathy hearkens back to longstanding traditions of valuing thought over feeling or reason over emotion. Today, however, new voices are being raised in praise of empathy and in opposition to the polarization, even dichotomization, of knowledge and affection, reason and emotion, professional detachment and compassionate care. This book presents a major new voice not only in the defense of empathy but in the expansion of its meanings and identification of guidelines for its development and practice.

Johanna Selles not only offers arguments in favor of empathy in human relationships, but also provides a rich descriptive analysis of the modes of empathy and an instructive, indeed inspiring, exploration of it as a response to human suffering. Here is no simplistic evaluation of experiences of empathy, and no simple formula for successful growth in empathic capacities. Here, rather, is a profound portrayal of empathic responses in multiple complex human contexts, and the gradual unfolding of criteria that can shape both empathy and its actions in constructive ways.

Combining concrete experiences with critical analysis, Selles exhibits as well as argues for the overcoming of false and unnecessary dichotomies in the responses of persons to human need. The book sometimes reads like a novel as much as like a theoretical and practical analysis. Its goal lies in the kind of insight that recognizes concrete human reality and responds with what might be called truthfulness in relationship—whether personal or professional. Hence, knowledge and emotion are mutually enhancing—loving knowledge and knowing love. And these concepts are treated in ways that defy any charges of sentimentalism or diminishment of professional discernment in action.

Of particular interest is the analysis of human suffering in both generic and specific forms. In some sense one might conclude accurately that for Selles (as for other sensitive students of humanity), "all suffering is the same." But of course it is not the same, as she would insist, if that means that a stock response to every form of suffering is sufficient. Selles takes into account concepts like "lament" and the diversity in experiences of pain, isolation, lostness in time. She provides a thought-provoking differentiation between personal suffering and suffering that is social (communal, cross-generational, or the suffering of particular groups). In a deeply moving chapter on bearing witness to human need and suffering, Selles shows the ways to transform what might be only pity into what she calls solidarity.

In opposition to some philosophers, Johanna Selles insists that virtue can be taught; at least empathy as a virtue can be learned and developed, shaping one's personality even in times of crisis. She turns creatively to describe possibilities of reflective, contemplative thinking, and pedagogies of imagination and transformation. Again, what is offered challenges and focuses thought and affection, so that it upbuilds even in its reading. Stages and contexts for learning are laid out with useful clarity, and their relevance not only for personal growth but for the development of empathic communities is persuasive and deeply moving.

Selles of course acknowledges the limits or dangers of empathy and the kind of high rhetoric without real insight that has given it a bad name in many traditions. She never overstates her case, and she asks for the kind of self-knowledge and self-discipline that sustain a focus on the one in need. This in turn, however, makes the empathic relationship mutually empowering, whether between caregiver and client, professional and patient, or one human being responding to the needs of another. Ultimately, Johanna Selles is reaching for wisdom in relationships—a kind of wisdom that can be shared between persons and may even generate communities of practice. This work goes a long way toward making this possible.

Margaret A. Farley
Yale University

Acknowledgments

THIS BOOK IS THE product of years of study, practice, and reflection with many empathic people. Although I cannot name them all here, I would like to acknowledge a few whose support was key to completing this book.

I am grateful to Professor Mary Molenwyk Doornbos and her colleagues for the invitation to participate in an event sponsored by the Calvin Center for Christian Scholarship. For me, the invitation was an opportunity to reflect on memories of nursing school and my first years of practice, which ultimately led to this project. Thanks to Otto Selles for editing and encouragement in that project.

And I am thankful for the opportunity to work at the Yale School of Nursing (2000–2002) as a nurse researcher on a project funded by the Patrick and Catherine Weldon Donaghue Medical Research Foundation. The Program for the Study of Health Care Relationships was a rich experience of reflection and collaboration on all aspects of the practitioner-client relationship. I would like to thank the principal investigators, Sally Cohen, Judith Krauss, and Regina Cusson, and the rest of the research team for the rich experiences at Yale in collaboration with the University of Connecticut. In addition, I thank my co-workers Sean Maher and Jeanetsey Velazquez.

I would like to acknowledge the inspiration and support of students, staff, and colleagues at Emmanuel College, Victoria University, Toronto School of Theology, and the University of Toronto. Family accompanied this project in emails, phone calls, and visits. I would like to thank my daughter Renata, a student in public health at Columbia University, as well as my niece, Johanna Ysselstein, a registered nurse at Toronto's Hospital for Sick Children, for the discussions and experiences we had together related to this topic.

During my research leave (2009–2010) I had the privilege of being a fellow at the Yale Interdisciplinary Center for Bioethics. I am grateful to Carol Pollard and David H. Smith, as well as other research fellows, board members, and staff for their challenging questions and keen interest in the subject. I was simultaneously a fellow at Yale Divinity School, and I am thankful to Dean Attridge and Paul Stuehrenberg for their hospitality. I would also like to acknowledge the kindness of Rev. Streets, Martha Smalley, the staff of Special Collections, and the students at YDS. Many thanks to Donna Diers for answering historical questions about Florence Wald. I thank Dr. Comer and Dr. Howard Spiro for agreeing to be interviewed for this project. Both continue to practice empathy and professional excellence in their respective remarkable careers.

Living in a cabin on a rock overlooking the tidal marsh of Long Island Sound from September to June 2010 was a strong reminder that reflection on suffering is best accompanied by observation of the beauty of the world. In addition, reuniting with old friends and meeting new ones made the year truly magnificent. Thanks especially to Nancy Thompson, Anne Howland, Karen Cheney, and Marilyn Anderson, Candace Taylor, as well as many others who, I hope, know how important they are and have been to this work. I would like to thank Christian Amondson of Wipf and Stock for supporting this project through all its stages of formation and Kristen Niehof for attention to editing detail.

I am grateful for past employment in patient care, research, clinical information systems, family health, education, and telemedicine, which exposed me to a variety of settings, such as a medical school (Yale School of Medicine); a nursing school (Yale School of Nursing); the Connecticut Hospice; Yale-New Haven Hospital; Northwest Regional Nurses' Agency; Public General Hospitals of Chatham and Sarnia, Ontario; Hospital for Sick Children, Toronto; and Boston University. The support of nursing colleagues, the good humor of staff, the wisdom of mentors, the courage of patients, and the tears and laughter that flourish in places such as a hospice are written into this project. Nurse friends over the years (thanks Linda and Hannah) have shared stories that directly influenced this book. I can only hope that the final product honors the work that continues in all these settings by those who practice empathic regard for themselves, their coworkers, and their clients.

Some of my learning precedes those professional experiences. I grew up in an immigrant household and community where my elders in an extended family shared the work of teaching, nursing, medicine, and clergy care. In retrospect, those tasks were less clearly delineated than professional schools might lead one to expect. The care of bodies (medicine), the nurture of souls (clergy) and the nurturance of learning and the heart (education) were housed under one roof in the presence of a minister father, teacher mother and doctor uncle. Furthermore, the presence in that household of my grandfather, an artist, left me with the conviction that creativity is at the very heart of empathy and might sustain professional practice in times of fatigue when empathy appears to have disappeared or while one waits for it to return. Even in those times, empathic communities can be built that sustain individual practitioners, clients, and communities in order that they can continue to work and educate for justice.

Introduction

IN THE ACCOUNT FROM the Gospel of John, Jesus visited Mary and Martha when he heard their brother was ill. By the time Jesus arrived, Lazarus had died. When he heard the news that Lazarus was dead, Jesus fully entered the sadness of the event and wept. If Jesus had been there as a professional student, he might have received some guidance on setting boundaries or avoiding excessive identification with a client. Jesus was there, however, as a friend who experienced the immanent and earthly reality of suffering, while drawing closer to his own death in the process.

Professionals in the helping professions face a variety of contradictions in their roles with clients. The rise of science as the preeminent paradigm for achieving health diminished the role of relationality in favor of instrumentality. The optimism that accompanied progress assumed that all could be fixed. Attention focused on those fixable things and ignored the unfixable. Past decades have attempted to correct these oversights by drawing our attention to the needs of chronic illness, the powerful witness of the differently abled, and the ever-present nature of poverty and marginalization.

Entering into another's sadness or joy "as if" it were our own can be regarded as evidence of emotional intelligence. The English language lacks precise language for such an ability. Sometimes called sympathy, compassion, or empathic engagement, the putting oneself in the "as if" situation requires skill, feeling, and imagination.

Although empathy is not a new idea, the notion that it might be a useful skill for therapeutic and professional relationships emerged in the nineteenth century. Since then, the idea of empathic engagement has found interested audiences in psychiatry, nursing, medicine, pastoral care, and teaching.

Beginning practitioners in those fields have likely absorbed mixed messages about experiencing or displaying empathic engagement with clients. In some cases, technical expertise or knowledge is privileged over the ability to intuit, feel, or imagine another's experience. But in other cases, empathy is seen as a useful technique or cognitive skill that can be practiced and learned to the benefit of the therapeutic relationship and its outcomes.

It is unfortunate that students in professional schools have few opportunities to share their experiences and learning in this area. Despite the lack of interprofessional dialogue, a growing awareness that caring too much may lead new practitioners into stress and burnout has created mentoring, group support, and teaching to help professionals manage their empathic engagement. In addition, schools that have prioritized scientific ways of knowing are beginning to acknowledge that some exposure to the humanities might improve professional practice.

This book intends to support the teaching and mentoring of professional students throughout their career by exploring the theoretical assumptions related to empathy. Although many of the tasks of clergy, teachers, nurses, and doctors can be effectively carried out without empathy, I will argue that empathic engagement is preferable, not only for the client, but also for the long-term nourishment of the professional life.

There are varying capacities for empathy that seem to be a product of one's character, nurture, experience, and valuing. These predispositions can be developed in professional education and experience, or they can be suppressed. Conversely, some individuals may have a low capacity for empathy and may need to engage in educational enhancements to encourage their ability to be empathic. If empathy were based solely on an emotional response, one could predict that certain professions or professional settings would quickly deplete one's ability to be empathic.

I practiced in a variety of clinical settings such as pediatrics, hospice, ICU-CCU, research, telemedicine, and psychiatry. I have trained and taught medical students, administrators, international students, nurses, religious educators, and students in professional ministry, formation, and social justice streams. Many students struggle with caring too much and bearing empathic burdens that at times threaten their professional formation. In one class called "Educating for Justice," students apply empathy to issues related to the environment, aboriginal issues, housing and homelessness, health care, poverty, and racism. Passionate engagement and empathic arousal does not always guarantee effective transmission of the ideas and feelings to others. In addition, liberal guilt easily slides into intolerance for those who see things differently. Working within diverse realities requires a high level of intercultural skill—empathy is an essential ingredient to that ability and to the ability to critique one's own privilege. Empathy is also useful to develop practices of reflection as one works in communities or organizations that may demand more from the individual practitioner than one can give.

I describe empathy as a two-stage process in relation to suffering: regarding suffering and acting or bearing witness in response to suffering. By exploring some of the pedagogy involved in educating for justice, students can be more aware of their experiences as they are educated in professional schools and their motivations for pursuing a profession. Much of professional practice involves teaching about care of the body, mind, and/or spirit of clients, their families and their communities. In this case, caring and empathy are not enough—it is also important to be self aware, contextually sensitive, and pedagogically astute.

In chapter 1, I examine current notions about professions and professional relationships in order to ascertain where empathy might fit. Chapter 2 studies the role of empathy in the therapeutic relationship and the difficulties of evaluating quantitative outcomes. Chapters 3 and 4 consider the two-step process of regarding suffering and bearing witness through action. Chapter 5 illustrates various types of educational interventions that might help to develop or shape empathic engagement. Chapter 6 looks at empathy as a resource for those who live and work in communities, whether in faith communities or NGOs, that work to improve the situations of others. In these various settings, I believe that empathy can make a difference that is mysterious and transcends our individual efforts. In making this claim, I realize I am putting empathy in a category with other mysterious and inexplicable concepts, such as love or creativity. Such concepts defy definition or empirical testing—however, most would agree that the world is a much better place with them than without.

It is my deep belief that professional practice is also better with empathy than without—both for the practitioner and for the client. The relationality that for aboriginal people around the world is the first principle of understanding has been slow to be appreciated in the world of science and progress. However, the plurality and the constant change that characterize the current workplace require a flexibility and creativity, as well as a spiritual grounding, that can sustain and improve the empathic abilities over time. The resulting mutuality and interconnectedness facilitates the professional relationship that seeks to treat one's neighbor, one's client, and the earth itself from a deep reservoir of empathy.

PART ONE

Theoretical Considerations

1

Professional Relationships

APPLYING TO BE A student at a professional school is a challenging experience involving transcripts, reference letters, resumes, statements of interest, application fees, and often evidence of volunteer work or research. The application process is only the first test—the second one involves surviving the demands of the program. This book serves as a guide to reflection on one aspect of professional formation, namely the ability to be empathic and to sustain empathic engagement in professional relationships. To begin, we will look at the following questions: *What is a profession? What is involved in the history of a profession? What is a professional relationship? What is empathy, and how does it affect the professional relationship?*

OBSERVING A PROFESSION

After she experienced some disabling headaches, Jill's friends convinced her that she needed to see a doctor. She made an appointment for a physical since she had never had a thorough check. On the day of her appointment, she leafed through magazines in the waiting room and watched the patients come and go in the office. She was eventually called into a small office and invited to take a seat. Her eyes wandered over the doctor's diploma from a nearby medical school, and then she noticed the examining table with a variety of instruments lined up. A blue gown was folded neatly on the table.

When Dr. Jones entered, she introduced herself and sat at the desk. While completing the history, the doctor asked Jill about the particular complaint that had led to the office visit, as well as her overall medical history. She left the room while Jill changed into the patient gown. During the physical assessment, Dr. Jones systematically checked and recorded data from her observations and continued to ask Jill questions related to her presenting complaint. Once Dr. Jones had completed the history and assessment, she wrote a prescription for medication and sent Jill to the laboratory for further blood work and urinalysis.

Although neither Jill nor Dr. Jones stopped to acknowledge the fact, their meeting was the beginning of a patient-practitioner relationship guided by unspoken rules and expectations. Jill quickly felt at ease with the professional setting of the clinic and with Dr. Jones's style, both of which balanced a caring attitude with a professional purpose. Dr. Jones recorded information in the patient chart. Jill was not worried that this information would be shared with others or used for inappropriate purposes. She assumed her chart would be filed and any subsequent lab results or notes would be added to that file.

During the appointment, Jill undressed and put on a patient gown. In any other setting, she would have felt very uncomfortable talking to a stranger in a state of relative undress. The setting and the doctor's professional attitude eased the awkwardness that Jill had initially felt while perched on the examining table with a small sheet and the blue gown for cover.

Both Jill and Dr. Jones operated in this encounter according to expectations that shape professional relationships. Each brought to the consultation a personal history and web of relationships that defined their expectations of health and illness. Primarily, though, their encounter was governed by unspoken expectations associated with a professional-client relationship involving respect, trust, safety, and confidentiality.

WHAT IS A PROFESSION?

The term "profession" was traditionally applied to law, medicine, and divinity—professions that traditionally excluded women until the late nineteenth and twentieth centuries. Arguments related to women's essential nature or social propriety were used to exclude women from professions and from science.[1] The story of women's entry and the entry of visible minorities into these professions is well documented elsewhere.[2] The entrance of women or visible minorities into professions did not,

1. Rossiter, *Women Scientists in America.*

2. See, for example, Hine, *Black Women in White* and Morantz-Sanchez, *Sympathy and Science.*

however, guarantee their full equality in the profession; many restrictions and limitations continued to be applied. Alternate forms of practice outside of the professional certification programs provided routes to practice for those still excluded from professional schools; discrimination against those alternative tracks continues to this day. In the nineteenth century, male doctors responded by using "science" to disqualify female lay healers and midwives.[3]

Entry into the historical learned professions assumed that a student had acquired a liberal education, including instruction in Latin or Greek. According to Gidney and Millar's study of professionals in nineteenth-century Upper Canada, professional status derived from social standing, liberal education, and membership in respectable classes, rather than from specific technical skills or knowledge.[4]

In modern times, professional status generally means that a person has completed postsecondary training including specialized skills, passed a certification test, and submitted to a degree of regulation by other practitioners.[5] Each profession tends to hold monopolistic control over its own work based on the specialized knowledge that distinguishes it from other forms of work.[6]

Professions change and adapt to the internal demands of their own professional associations, as well to external demands from society or government. Educational changes in a professional school can include higher admission standards, increased practical experience or required clinical hours, or a shift in the form of curriculum evaluation, such as outcomes-based assessment. An example of one such potential shift can be found in a recent report on nursing that recommends that nurses obtain a master's degree within ten years of graduation from a baccalaureate.[7] Resistance to such changes may derive from the institutions, faculty, or students.

The reality gap between professional education and the practice setting can sometimes become uncomfortably large in two opposite ways: teachers who were trained in another era may continue to teach as they were taught, or teachers may introduce innovations that are too

---

3. Code, *What Can She Know?* 226.

4. Gidney and Millar, *Professional Gentlemen*, 5.

5. Kinnear, *In Subordination*, 7.

6. Freidson, *Professionalism*, 30–31.

7. Benner et al., *Educating Nurses*.

advanced for the daily realities of the practice setting. Some professional schools attempt to overcome these gaps by requiring that faculty retain one foot in the clinical/practice setting. The rate of change in those settings, accelerated by the use of technology, creates uncertainty for students as they struggle to master knowledge that will likely be outdated before they graduate. Although attempts have been made in a variety of disciplines to disseminate research findings or transfer knowledge more rapidly, the lag between new knowledge and teaching remains difficult to overcome. Demands for research dissemination are now increasingly heard in the humanities; individuals and institutions seek to adopt models of relevance and change to a body of knowledge that once had been considered to be essential and unchanging.

SCIENCE VERSUS HUMANITIES

The growing and virtually unquestioned predominance of science as the exclusive basis for knowledge and method in modern times has created a separation among professional education programs. Although doctors and clergy shared a classical liberal curriculum in the nineteenth century, the rise of specialized professional training programs without a humanities core resulted in a fracture between the sciences and the humanities. The educated gentleman doctor had less and less in common with educated clergy—a rationalized division of labor made one a specialist in the body and the other in the soul. In this way, the science-based curriculum made exclusive claims on its adherents that gradually devalued other types of knowledge and other ways of knowing. Current attempts to overcome the fracture through programs in Humanities in Medicine provide a creative challenge to an otherwise dominant scientific paradigm.

Nineteenth-century students of nursing and teaching were educated in programs housed in hospital-based schools of nursing and in normal schools and teacher-training programs. As these programs pushed upward into baccalaureate streams, they still occupied separate classrooms and methods, with science increasingly the sole authority for nursing knowledge and practice. Pre-baccalaureate nursing programs focused on the clinical divisions such as medical-surgical, obstetrics, and others, with one additional course focused on the humanities of nursing. The notion of independent nursing research was not part of the professional development of the diploma nurse; current university-based nursing makes nursing research essential.

Most professional programs undergo shifts over time in emphases and curriculum. Clergy training, for example, increasingly values specialized learning and skills that can be measured and evaluated, shifting to a uniformity that has more in common with technocratic culture and technical training models.[8] In addition, faith communities demand multiskilled practitioners, where once proclamation and interpretation of text were the preeminent abilities. Although in past decades faith communities were able to engage professional staff with separate specializations in pastoral care, education, or preaching, current economic realities often demand that clergy function in all these areas with equal competence and in multiple sites.

PROFESSIONAL BEHAVIOR

Professional behavior may include independent thinking, creativity, ability to work collaboratively, leadership, and organizational skills. Other skills might include the ability to communicate effectively, show initiative, and use sound clinical reasoning or judgment. Professionals may be expected to have or to acquire a degree of social intelligence or relational abilities, including self-awareness, skills in conflict management, and the ability to accept criticism.

Not all professional training programs value relational capacities equally—work settings that place a high value on technical and research competencies place less emphasis on social skills; indeed, some forms of professional care can deliver positive outcomes for the client without a high degree of relationality. Sometimes the emotional care of the client falls by default to an auxiliary professional group. Lorraine Code observes that doctors have been associated with knowledge, as opposed to nurses, who are linked with experience. The division of labor that results allows the doctor to treat the patient's condition with professional effectiveness, whereas compassion becomes the exclusive domain of the nurse.[9] As professional nurses become increasingly involved in case management, the caring tasks may default to nursing assistants or other auxiliary staff. The intersubjective abilities that are often assumed to be

8. Cherry, *Hurrying toward Zion.*
9. Code, *What Can She Know?* 222.

part of the professional ethos are challenging to identify, name, evaluate, and teach (see chapter 5 for more on educating for empathy).

WHAT IS A PROFESSIONAL RELATIONSHIP?

A professional relationship differs from a personal relationship. An individual might, however, have a personal relationship with someone who also functions as a practitioner, such as a teacher or clergyperson. When a professional has more than one role, the professional is described as being in a dual relationship. These relationships can function without any problem over time, as long as both participants honor boundaries and respect confidentiality.

For the purposes of this discussion, however, the professional-client relationship assumes a client who seeks a particular type of service that is offered by the professional, who is a stranger. This relationship may take the following forms: teacher-learner, practitioner-patient, clergy-client, or nurse-patient. There are many other professionals who engage in a professional relationship, including licensed massage therapists, physiotherapists, occupational therapists, naturopaths, nutritionists, art therapists, and others.

The referral that may originate from yet another professional results in a consultation, during which information is exchanged and a plan is established. The consultation may be a onetime event or part of an ongoing professional relationship. At all times this relationship is governed by both ethical standards and technical competencies that have been part of the professional's training and continue to be the focus of postgraduate continuing education.

THE DYAD

The professional relationship is generally depicted as a dyad in the medical literature. The dyad is a theoretical simplification—in practice, the client brings to the consultation a complex set of relationships with partners, relatives, and the community. The professional also represents a network of relationships related to family or other affiliations that inform professional life. A nurse whispers to his colleague that he feels somewhat dizzy due to fasting for Ramadan; a resident yawns with fatigue as a result of being on call while being a new mother to twins. These external relationships are not physically part of the dyad but still exert an influence on the daily life of a professional. Professionalism demands that one provide quality standards of care irrespective of any challenges in one's personal life. Professional self-care demands that the professional monitor and seek help when personal demands undermine professional excellence. A lack of self-care will deplete the empathic abilities.

Several generalizations can be made about the professional relationship. The dyad or client-practitioner relationship has generally been understood as a functional entity that results in positive outcomes for treatment. Based on this functional interpretation, education for the professional attempts to improve the professional's relational skills in order to ensure these beneficial outcomes for the client. The professional relationship can also be viewed as having a high degree of mutuality, wherein the client has an important role in sharing information and making decisions. Information available on the Internet facilitates another model: the client as a consumer who arrives at the consultation with information and options. A third model of the relationship allows the professional to function as an expert, with a passive and uninformed client. Educational assumptions for this type of professional relationship stress the skill and expertise of the professional.

Each profession has its own language to describe aspects of professional relationship. In a study of pastoral care, Dayringer defines the therapeutic relationship as "the spontaneous and earned reciprocity of affective attitudes that persons hold toward each other."[10] Nursing standards describe the components of the nurse-client therapeutic relationship as containing power, trust, respect, and intimacy: "based on trust, respect, and intimacy with the client, the relationship also requires the appropriate use of power."[11] The teacher-learner relationship also values respect and trust. Often depicted in movies, the teacher-student relationship has been portrayed as a powerful force for change.

TRUST AND ETHICS

Each profession has a code of ethics and practice guidelines that are continually revised to meet new conditions of practice. The rules that shape a professional relationship vary greatly from profession to profession. Clients assume that their practitioners will operate from within those

10. Dayringer, *Heart of Pastoral Counseling*, 3.
11. "Standards for the Therapeutic Nurse-Client Relationship."

rules. Violation of that trust can be a devastating experience for clients. Appropriate boundaries for each profession may vary; for example, a health care professional may be required to touch a patient's body in ways that would be inappropriate for other professionals, but necessary for the therapeutic outcomes of the relationship in the health care setting.[12]

The professional relationship is governed by ethical standards, a subject that is increasingly represented in the professional curriculum. Coutts observes that health care ethics became more prominent in the medical curriculum during the late 1960s, when several medical schools established ethics teaching in their medical curricula. Ethics, it was felt, would provide the humanities component and equip doctors for the increasing complexity of medical decision making.[13] A survey of United States' medical schools in 1979 revealed that of the 107 schools that responded, 97 indicated that they taught some type of medical ethics. This teaching ranged from special lectures on the topic, or electives in the area (47 schools), whereas required courses were only offered at six of the schools. Between 1972 and 1979, the faculties of medicine with a commitment to teaching ethics increased by 50 percent.[14]

WHAT IS EMPATHY?

As a manifestation of emotional intelligence, empathy is increasingly part of the mission of professional education. Definitions of empathy often highlight the capacity for understanding and sharing another's feelings or ideas. In addition, empathy is often characterized as the ability to put oneself in another's shoes "as if" they were one's own. The ability to experience the "as if" requires a degree of emotional resonance. The question remains, is such emotional resonance a cognitive skill or an affective capacity? Second, if this skill is an essential component of client-practitioner relationships, can it be learned?

Although the term was adopted from the German language, the capacity for empathy has presumably been present in human encounters since the earliest times. Empathy allows two or more persons to cooperate in a variety of social functions. In being able to cooperate and create a sustainable society, or in being able to predict and defeat

---

12. Benner, *From Novice to Expert.*

13. Coutts, "Teaching Ethics in the Health Care Setting."

14. Veatch and Sollitto, "Medical Ethics Teaching," 1030–33.

an enemy, the capacity for empathy might thus be considered an essential human skill.

Some ambivalence about the importance of empathy continues to exist; empathy can be seen as something that threatens professional judgment or something that can improve intuition or diagnostic abilities. Empathy has been used to understand individual behavior, social behavior, and creative behavior. For professionals, empathy is increasingly seen as a valuable resource that enhances both the professional relationship and the outcomes of that encounter. Less frequently, empathy is understood as a mutually experienced aspect of the professional relationship that can help regenerate the ability to care, both for the professional and for the client-other.

THE MEANING OF THE TERM

The origin of the word "empathy" can be traced from the Greek *empatheia*, literally meaning passion (*empathes*), and from feelings and emotion (em + pathos)—appreciation of the feelings of the other. Empathy has been defined as the power of projecting one's personality into the object of contemplation, and so fully understanding it.[15]

Although the term was claimed by a variety of disciplines, including biblical hermeneutics, the origin of the concept is generally traced to the late nineteenth century as part of the psychology of aesthetics. At that time, *Einfühlung* described the tendency of observers to project themselves into that which they observed. Nineteenth-century German philosopher of aesthetics Robert Vischer used the term *Einfühlung* in 1873 to describe the emotional response felt by an observer when regarding a work of art. *Einfühlung* ("feeling-into") had a different sense than sympathy, or "feeling-with." These ideas were rooted in the philosopher Kant's idea that the beauty of an object was grounded in the observer, as opposed to the object itself.

At the end of the nineteenth century, Theodore Lipps applied the term *Einfühlung* to the discipline of psychology. Lipps described his sense of watching a circus performer and feeling as if he were inside him. According to Halpern, his definition referred to an experiential type of knowing that is essentially affective. She notes that the phrase "projecting

---

15. Spiro et al., eds., *Empathy and the Practice of Medicine.*

one's personality" refers to the experience of connection between one's own affective condition and the object one is trying to understand.[16]

In 1903 William Wundt transferred the term to human relationships, and shortly thereafter Sigmund Freud used *Einfühlung* to describe "the psychodynamics of putting oneself in another person's position."[17] Edward Titchener, a Cornell psychologist who was able to translate the German tradition to Americans, invented the English word "empathy" as a translation of Lipps's *Einfuhlung* and used the term to suggest "understanding" of other human beings.[18]

Southard, in the early twentieth century, observed that empathy was significant in facilitating diagnostic outcomes in a therapeutic relationship. Since these early theorists, empathy has found its way into psychotherapeutic and counseling literature, as well as other fields, such as teaching and social work.[19]

A variety of disciplines claim empathy as an essential trait. Philosopher Martin Buber (1878–1965) described empathy as a state of being as experienced by another in dialogue.[20] He believed that our access to being comes through "our capacity to enter into dialogue or relationship with the existent, or the between." Buber described humans as being capable of entering relationships with each other that have a transcendent capacity and are defined as "I-thou" relations; by contrast, the "I-it" relationship sees the other as a tool. Buber described a quality of presence that allows one to be totally in tune with the other.[21]

Empathy also has roots in hermeneutics. Ellen Singer More notes that empathy entered the modern critical tradition through the hermeneutical tradition of *verstehen*, or "understanding." More describes this as an extension of the nineteenth-century biblical interpretation developed by Schleiermacher, Dilthey, and Weber.[22]

Modell traces the origins of empathy even earlier to the notion of self entering the object of perception described by Vico (1668–1744),

---

16. Halpern, *From Detached Concern*, 75.

17. Hojat, *Empathy in Patient Care*, 4.

18. More and Milligan, eds., *Empathic Practitioner*, 21.

19. Hojat, *Empathy in Patient Care*, 5.

20. Buber, *I and Thou*, 46.

21. DeWitt Baldwin, "Philosophical and Psychological Contributions," 39–60.

22. More and Milligan, eds., *Empathic Practitioner*.

who believed that "meaning is constructed through imaginatively enter-ing into the minds of others."[23]

EMPATHY AND SYMPATHY

Although some definitions attempt to distinguish between empathy and sympathy, in reality, the distinctions are unclear. In empathy, observers imagine the experience of another "as if" the experience were their own, whereas sympathy suggests that the observer is absorbed or immersed in feeling all the experiences of the other, sometimes resulting in a feel-ing of pity for the person. Educator and writer Brené Brown defines em-pathy as a skill that allows one to connect with the experience of another. She argues that part of that skill involves tapping into one's own experi-ences. Compassion is the willingness to be open to that process as equals in a relationship. From extensive research, Brown argues that sympathy results in distance and disconnection, with a marked separation between the observer and the observed. Empathy, by contrast, results in connec-tion and relationship through the practice of nonjudgmental listening.[24]

In a concept analysis of the term, nursing professor Theresa Wiseman notes the absence of a clear working definition of sympathy. Wiseman concludes her concept analysis by highlighting four aspects of empathy, including: (1) the ability to listen, (2) the ability to take on another's term of reference, (3) the ability to understand and not judge, and (4) the ability to communicate that understanding.[25] Her review of the literature supports the idea that a person may have a disposition to be empathic (trait), but whether one actually is empathic depends on a number of factors (state). The implications for educators are clear: if empathy is considered an essential trait, one might attempt to select students with a predisposition to empathy; but because it is also a state, educators need to be mindful of the way the educational process sup-ports, enhances, or inhibits the ability to be empathic.

Part of the confusion is a result of the different development of the terms and their adoption by a variety of disciplines. Sympathy emerged with the eighteenth-century economic theory of Adam Smith. Smith believed humans could experience a "fellow feeling" when they observed

23. Modell, *Imagination and the Meaningful Brain*, 118.

24. Brown, *I Thought It Was Just Me*, 33–50.

25. Wiseman, "Concept Analysis," 1162–67.

someone experiencing a powerful emotion; the resulting feelings might include pity, anguish, or joy. Smith called this affective state sympathy—an emotion triggered by the power of the imagination.[26] This sympathetic state allows one to experience sensations similar to, but weaker than, those experienced by another person.

Herbert Spencer's *Principles of Psychology* (1870) argued that humans affiliate with others of their species to adapt and provide safety. Over time humans developed pleasure from affiliation. A high level of social contact allows sympathy to develop as a result of repeated association. For Spencer, sympathy is largely a means of communication.[27] McDougall's 1908 *Introduction to Social Psychology* claimed that sympathy focuses on how the target and observer share emotional reactions. He believed that sympathetic reactions were the result of built-in perceptual mechanisms.[28]

The imprecision of the term "empathy" is further confused by its close relationship to similar terms such as compassion, caring, pity, as well as confusion generated by translation from French and German to English. Stotland distinguishes empathy from sympathy by the observation that empathy is more active. In empathy, one attends to the feelings of another, whereas in sympathy, one attends to the suffering of another, but the feelings are one's own. Stotland defines empathy in the following way: "An observer reacting emotionally because he perceives that another is experiencing or about to experience an emotion." In this definition, the meaning, measurement, and direction of the emotion are important and exclude both *projection* (I attribute my emotions to the other) and *labeling* (I use the other to define my own reactions). My empathic reaction may involve similar feelings to the person I am observing, but the feelings will rarely be exactly the same. A variety of factors, including my own history and personality, will affect what I see.[29] According to this theory, one can approximate the emotional responses of the other, but the layers of individual interpretation and experience always provide variation.

---

26. Davis, *Empathy*, chapter 2.
27. Spencer, *Principles of Psychology*.
28. McDougall, *Introduction to Social Psychology*, 3–4.
29. Stotland et al., *Empathy*, 8.

EMPATHY AND PSYCHOANALYTIC THEORY

Carl Rogers (1902–1987), the founder of client-centered therapy, suggested empathy as a way of relating interpersonally for the purpose of the collaborative work of healing. Rogers described empathy as an ability to perceive the internal frame of reference of another with accuracy, as if one were the other person, but without ever losing the "as if" condition. Professionals might strive for a state of acceptance of their clients, which Rogers called unconditional positive regard. For Rogers, this capacity involved cognitive understanding rather than emotional involvement. Rogers noted that when he was intensely focused on the client, "just my presence seems to be healing."[30] Some schools of psychoanalytic theory stress the affective quality of the process, "which is viewed as a consequence of the mechanism of identification as delineated by Freud." Fenichel described two steps to the process: (1) identification with the other person, and (2) awareness of one's own feelings after the identification as well as an awareness of the object's feelings.[31]

EMPATHY AS A MODE OF UNDERSTANDING

Psychoanalyst Heinz Kohut (1913–1987) described empathy as a mode of cognition that is specifically attuned to the perception of a complex psychological configuration. Kohut was doubtful that empathy could generate positive effects for the patient-practitioner relationship because he believed that empathy could not by itself be perceived as supportive or therapeutic; rather, it was a precondition to being supportive or therapeutic. In other words, even if a mother's empathy toward her child is correct and accurate, it is not her empathy that satisfies her child's needs. Her actions and responses to the child do this.[32] Kohut used empathy as an "information gathering activity" that allowed him to formulate an "experience near" model of the client's inner dynamics and subsequently use empathy as a treatment tool. Empathy, defined as "vicarious introspection," meant that only through introspection into one's own experience could one learn what it might be like for another person in a similar experience. Steps involved in this empathy include introspection into oneself and then vicarious introspection into another (that is, empathy),

30. Michele Baldwin, *Use of Self in Therapy*, 45.

31. Fenichel, *Psychoanalytic Theory of Neurosis*, 511.

32. Kohut, *Analysis of the Self*, 300.

which allows one to observe a person's inner life, including thoughts, ideas, and mental states.[33]

EMPATHY AND SOCIAL INTELLIGENCE— COGNITIVE APPROACHES

Philosopher and sociologist George Herbert Mead (1863–1931) described empathy as the capacity to take the role of another person and adopt alternative perspectives. Empathy involves accuracy in predicting another's thoughts or feelings. According to Mead, social behavior begins when one learns by means of interacting with others that one exists separately.[34] In his study of Mead, Keith (2009) notes that awareness of the self makes possible the empathic connection with others in society. We take on the attitude of the other, and consequently, "it is the capacity for empathy that grounds the realization that we evolve out of social and natural relationships and that we, in turn, shape those environments."[35] The ability to put oneself in the role of the other gives rise to the ethical self. Mead was the first to describe empathy as an element of social intelligence—a theme that anticipates the writing of Salovey and Mayer (1990) and of Goleman (1995), who describe empathy as a domain of emotional intelligence.

EMPATHY AND CHILD DEVELOPMENT

Psychiatrist Harry Stack Sullivan (1892–1949) viewed empathy as important in infant development prior to speech. Sullivan noted that tension in a mother creates anxiety in the child. He attributed this to an interpersonal process that he described as empathy. Concerning this process Sullivan wrote the following:

> But whether the doctrine of empathy is accepted or not, the fact remains that the tension of anxiety when present in the mothering one induces anxiety in the infant; that theorem can be proved; I believe, and those who have had pediatric experience or mothering experience actually have data which can be interpreted on no other equally simple hypothetical basis. So although empathy may sound mysterious, remember that there is much that sounds

33. MacIssac, "Empathy," 245–64.

34. Mead, *Mind, Self, and Society*, 135.

35. Keith, "Transforming Ren," 69–84.

mysterious in the universe, only you have got used to it; and perhaps you will get used to empathy.[36]

Modern child development and cognitive psychologists are more indebted to Piaget when they see empathy as a form of social cognition or a mature or non-egocentric stage in the process of cognitive development. Empathy is more than merely understanding another's feelings—it involves a deeper understanding.[37]

THERAPEUTIC EMPATHY

Christian Huygens (1629–1695) observed that when two clocks were mounted on a common support, they would beat in unison—a principle he named *entrainement*. Sometimes translated as "resonance," this principle, when applied to a professional relationship, suggests that strangers can learn to practice deep listening and emerge with a quality of resonance. Therapeutic empathy involves taking the perspective of the client. By communicating a perception of the client's situation, the therapist displays empathy, and that skill enables the therapist to assume the perspective of the client. The following three skills are prerequisites to empathy: identifying emotions in oneself and others; assuming the perspective of others; and expressing emotion in a controlled, articulate manner.[38]

Code notes that empathy opens up conversation and includes self-reflexive skills that "enables its practitioners to judge the kind and degree of empathy a situation, a person, or a group requires: and to hold back at places where their habitual empathic practices may be inappropriate, excessive, or inadequate."[39]

In an excellent study of empathy, Halpern offers a model for therapeutic empathy that rejects both extremes of detached insight and affective merging. She relies on resonance, which allows the practitioner to use the imagination as a framework for understanding the patient's experience. Theories of empathy fall in two traditions of the patient-physician relationship: those that emphasize detached knowledge and those that emphasize sympathy. Halpern argues that empathy requires

36. Sullivan, *Interpersonal Theory of Psychiatry*, 41–42.

37. Craig, *Philosophical and Educational Foundations*, chapter 3.

38. Feshbach, "Empathy," 33–59.

39. Code, "I Know Just How You Feel," 77–97.

experiential, not just theoretical, knowing. She believes empathy resembles hypothesizing. The kind of knowledge involved in empathy depends on cognitive knowledge, as well as imagination. Although resonance contributes to empathy, it is not sufficient for grasping another's distinct emotional perspective and requires cognitive engagement.[40]

Neurobiology contributes exciting new insights into empathy. Mirror neurons in the brain facilitate connections between the experiencer and the observer.[41] The shared neural activation pattern can thus provide a biological basis for understanding another person's mind.[42]

COGNITIVE VERSUS AFFECTIVE

Debates continue about whether empathy is a cognitive or affective attribute or a combination. Bennett describes empathy as containing both aspects when he describes it as a "mode of relating in which one person comes to know the mental content of another, both affective and cognitive, at a particular moment in time and as a product of the relationship that exists between them."[43]

Hojat differentiates between reasoning and appraisal (part of cognitive responses) and spontaneity and arousal (the hallmarks of emotional responses). If this definition holds true, then the cognitive part of empathy relies more on learning and advanced reasoning, whereas the affective part is more effortless, spontaneous, and primitive.[44]

MUTUALITY AND POWER

Empathy can provide a way to approach difference and interact meaningfully with the other. Huffaker argues that little attention has been paid to how the experience of "holding otherness" contributes to the development of human selfhood. Everding and Huffaker define empathy as "one's ability to take the role of another in order to understand the other's feelings, perspectives, and ideas." On the basis of their research on development and identity formation, they conclude that "what dis-

40. Halpern, *From Detached Concern*, chapter 4.

41. See, for example, Modell, *Imagination and the Meaningful Brain*.

42. Gallese, "Intentional Attunement," 131–75.

43. Bennett, ed., *Empathic Healer*, 2.

44. Hojat, *Empathy in Patient Care*, 7–10.

tinguishes relationships that nurture selfhood and clarify identity is their mutuality of empathy."[45]

Mutuality in relationship improves the ability to express empathy and to respond to the inner world of the other.[46] The professional can make an ongoing commitment to attempt to see the world from the perspective of those who are generally marginalized or subjugated. Such a contextual analysis relies on understanding not only the individual patient/client, but also includes the social context that contributes to the client's situation.

Empathy cannot be understood without a focus on power. There are many distortions of empathy that result from disregarding the power relations in the therapeutic relationship. Empathy in a professional or therapeutic relationship can be either caring and supportive or intrusive and coercive. In the patient-practitioner relationship, the practitioner might assume what a person feels or presume to tell people what they are feeling. In both cases, the practitioner is assuming power over the patient. Empathy has negative potential when a practitioner uses knowledge of other people to control or manipulate them.[47]

Candib defines empathy as "the readiness to feel the other's feelings as one's own and to use that awareness for the benefit of the other." Empathy is a precondition for empowerment because through empathy "the person knows she has been heard, felt, touched." Empathy consists of engrossment (apprehending the other's reality) and inclusion (the one caring practices confirmation).[48]

Responding to the other requires a flexibility that runs counter to scientific practice, which generally depends on repeatability under controlled conditions. Ruddick's work on mothering as a model prioritizes skills of innovation, disclosure, and responsiveness instead of clarity and certainty. By contrast with the replicability of science, maternal thinking responds to constant change.[49] A professional prepared to respond to change and complexity requires different skills than practitioners of another era, who were outfitted with skills and enduring knowledge that were not expected to change.

---

45. Huffaker, *Creative Dwelling*, 46–47.

46. Jordan, ed., *Women's Growth in Diversity.*

47. Code, "I Know Just How You Feel," 77–97.

48. Candib, "Reconsidering Power," 135–56.

49. Ruddick, "Maternal Thinking," 213–30.

PROFESSIONAL SCHOOLS AND EMPATHY

Many professional schools would agree that one of the goals of professional and postprofessional education is the formation of an empathic practitioner. How can the curriculum, both explicit and implicit, intentionally produce practitioners with desirable interpersonal skills and empathic abilities? Can this relational ability be taught, mentored, encouraged, and developed, or is this ability resident (or absent) in the individual and unlikely to be affected by any type of pedagogy or curriculum? The notion of professional formation includes not only skills and knowledge, but also the attitudes that allow one to be empathic towards the self and other in the course of one's professional career. In an implicit curriculum that emphasizes the privilege derived from specialized knowledge, how can a culture of mutuality and empathy be valued and promoted? The next chapter will look at the practitioner-client relationship in health care as one example of this professional relationship. The challenges of attempting to isolate a relational variable in the professional relationship will also be explored.

SUMMARY

Definitions of the term empathy are complex and contradictory and owe their imprecision to the influence of a variety of disciplines, including sociology, psychology, economics, biblical hermeneutics, and psychoanalysis. Sympathy is often distinguished from empathy as feeling sorry for a person or imagining how one would feel in the same situation, whereas empathy demands that one imagines what it is like being that person and experiencing things as they do. [50] For the purposes of this work, empathy will be described as a trait that has affective and cognitive components that can be enhanced or diminished through educational experiences that can contribute to the professional relationship and the development of mutuality and connection.

Many contemporary writers agree that empathy has an "as if" quality of perception of the other that relies on both cognitive and affective elements. Professional schools generally value empathy as a desirable trait for the professional to bring to the therapeutic relationship. Questions remain—how can one identify this trait; how can one teach students to

---

50. Wiseman, "Concept Analysis," 1164.

achieve it; how can it be evaluated; and what types of curricular experiences support empathy?

To return to the opening scenario of Jill and Dr. Jones, Jill left the doctor's office relieved that the doctor had heard her complaints, prescribed medicine, and promised follow-up on the laboratory examinations. The doctor had fulfilled her professional obligations to diagnose, treat, listen, and attempt to cure or relieve symptoms using the technical and scientific knowledge that she had acquired in her training. But there was an aspect of the encounter that was more difficult to describe or measure, but that influenced Jill's overall satisfaction with the encounter. Jill felt that her new doctor had been empathic, and she felt relieved that Dr. Jones had seemed to understand how painful and debilitating her migraine headaches were. No one in her family seemed to take her headaches seriously—in fact, they were very impatient with Jill when she could not get out of bed to go to work.

Although Dr. Jones had never personally experienced a migraine, she was able to put herself in Jill's shoes and imagine "as if" she were the patient. Was her ability to do this a learned skill, or was it merely an expression of the caring personality that had led her to apply to medical school in the first place? Did her medical studies and clinical experiences increase or decrease her ability to be empathic? Would Dr. Jones sustain this ability over the course of her career, or would she gradually lose the ability to imagine herself in the shoes of her patients?

From the perspective of Dr. Jones, did the ability to imagine Jill's headaches exacerbate the stress of her own day, or did the empathic connection energize her work? Was this encounter affected by the ethnicity, race, class, or religious background of the client and the practitioner? And finally, could any of these factors be isolated, examined, and quantified in an empirical study allowing the control of a factor that could be called a "relational" factor or "empathic capacity" in the study?

QUESTIONS FOR FURTHER REFLECTION

1. Describe the history of the founding of your professional school. Was it affiliated with a university or college? Who were the founders? How was the school funded?

2. Find a description of the required courses or curriculum for the early years of the school. How does it compare to your own curriculum?

3. Were there any social traditions, student societies, or professional organizations associated with the school? Compare these to your current experience of student life.

4. Locate a primary source document related to the history of the school. If you can photocopy this document, do so. Create some questions to ask of the document. Once you have created a series of questions, try to write answers to these questions. Match up the questions to any resources you can find: for example, a history of the school or an account of the student experience by an alumnus. Photographs, architectural plans, lecture notes, speeches, convocation addresses, and sermons can all provide useful insights into the history of your professional school.

5. Find an alumnus of the program to interview, either in person or through previously published biographical files or journal articles. Compare the person's experience to your own.

6. Write a review of a book that describes the history of your profession.

7. Have you recently been in a professional relationship as either the client or the practitioner? Do you think empathy was involved in the interaction? Describe the places where you think empathy was present. Do you think of that relationship as therapeutic?

8. Does your professional school mention empathy in its mission statement? Or other words such as compassion or care? How do you think those concepts are being or have been taught?

2

The Health-Care Relationship

The Roots of Therapeutic Empathy

M Y PATIENT, A WOMAN in her thirties, was five months pregnant. She had been admitted to intensive care with a pulmonary embolism and was being treated with medications to thin her blood. However, the medication was posing a risk to her pregnancy. During the night she went into premature labor and delivered in the early morning. The patient asked us, the two night nurses, to perform a baptism. The small hospital had no clergy on call during the night shift. Despite feeling unprepared for the task, we wanted to honor the patient's request. That night, while the other patients slept, we baptized the child and wept quietly in the utility room of the dimly lit intensive care unit.

We might have refused or told the patient to wait until daytime, when the pastoral staff would be available. We could have said that we were not trained to do religious rituals. That night, though, unschooled in liturgical practices and feeling completely inadequate to the task, we did our best to provide the patient with empathy and spiritual care.

When I returned to check on the patient, she took my hand and said, "I hope this experience will not discourage you from someday having children." I was stunned that even in the midst of her loss, the patient was reaching out to comfort me. Her capacity for empathy in the midst of personal loss left a deep impression on me.

INTRODUCTION

In the previous chapter, I examined the professional relationship and the role of empathy. The health-care relationship is one of the most studied versions of the professional relationship. This chapter will focus on the health-care relationship, to gain insight into the complexity of attempting to quantify empathy or relational variables in a professional relationship.

The health-care dyad has been studied in terms of the events leading up to the consultation (health-seeking behaviors, client expectations, referral patterns); the nature of the consultation (communication studies, models of practitioner behavior); and the results or outcomes of the consultation (adherence, patient satisfaction). Studies have examined the health-care relationship in terms of the progression of disease (acute, chronic); disease types (diabetes, hypertension); the notion of trust or affiliation; and organizational factors that affect care.

What can we learn from the way the therapeutic relationship has been described and studied? How does empathy fit that relationship? What are the boundaries of therapeutic empathy? What can other professions learn from the literature and research on the health-care relationship?

PRIOR TO THE ENCOUNTER

As described in chapter 1, the health-care encounter is often described as a dyad consisting of the client and the practitioner (who might be a doctor, nurse, psychiatrist, psychologist, social worker, or other health professional). This dyad is governed by professional standards of behavior; client expectations; cultural, religious, and ethnic factors; gender expectations; and a host of unspoken and unseen factors. The encounter might be a onetime event (for acute problems) or a continuing series of encounters (for chronic conditions).

For a professional student, the encounter can generate anxiety as the student hopes to present a professional and competent exterior while tackling new skills. Mentors review clinical settings and review conversations with students before and after such encounters in order to help them reflect on the encounter. Clinical instructors are generally alert to situations in which students are overly involved with patients and demonstrate excessive empathy, or empathic overload. On the other hand, students who seem devoid of empathic concern might be of concern to an instructor as well. The value instructors place on students' empathic abilities varies with how they view the nature of the health-care relationship and the role of relationality in achieving positive outcomes.

MODELS OF THE HEALTH-CARE RELATIONSHIP

Within the dyad of patient-practitioner, the relationship can take different forms. Szasz and Hollander describe three models of the doctor-patient relationship: activity-passivity, guidance-cooperation, and mutual participation. Models of relationship can have implications for the definition, treatment, and therapeutic outcomes of illness. The ideal model for relationship in health care involves mutual participation, in which the doctor helps the patient to help him- or herself and the patient works in partnership with the doctor, allowing both to occupy adult roles and to work together.[1]

Terms used to describe the health-care relationship include mutuality, partnership, respect, autonomy, shared decision-making, and power sharing. In recent decades the traditional model of the health-care relationship has changed due to the growth of the empowerment model, increased diversity of the population, diversification of health-care practitioners, the rise of the consumer model, and increased management of care. The traditional biomedical model in medical relationships traditionally assumed a paternalistic doctor and an obedient patient; current models of the relationship have shifted to a bio-psychosocial model that attempts to include the complexity of the patient's socio-economic background, gender, race, and cultural background.

A shift from a paternalistic model to a decision-sharing model is a radical change for a professional relationship that has been based for centuries on the unquestioned authority of the physician.[2] Despite this new shift, little information is available on how this changed relationship affects the patient experience of health-care outcomes. Education alone may be insufficient to shift the paradigm adequately to allow patients to take an active role in self-management of their conditions or to transform all clinicians into flexible, shared decision-making practitioners. Some patients may even prefer a traditional hierarchical relationship.

Nursing literature has demonstrated a consistent interest in the nurse-patient health-care relationship. Travelbee describes the nursing relationship as one that passes through stages—beginning with the phase of original encounter and evolving to the phase of rapport.[3] Nursing

---

1. Szasz and Hollander, "Contribution to the Philosophy of Medicine," 585–92.
2. Katz, *Silent World of Doctor and Patient*.
3. Travelbee, *Interpersonal Aspects of Nursing*.

theorists generally agree that communication is central to the nurse's work. The purpose of the nurse-patient relationship is to help patients accept and find meaning in their experiences or to accept their humanity, which leads to hope.[4] Nursing theorists including Virginia Henderson, Lydia Hall, Jean Watson, Patricia Benner, Dorothy Orem, Martha Rogers, Dorothy Johnson, and Sister Callista Roy have contributed to a body of theory that seeks to place the nurse-patient relationship at the center of nursing practice.[5] According to many of these nursing theorists, the goals of the health-care relationship include the co-construction of meaning; the return or maintenance of self-care of the client; the setting of goals with a client; the process of caring; and the return to balance, harmony, or healing. Nursing theorists also place caring on a continuum from those who believe that professional detachment is the most effective model to those who feel that an intense personal relationship is key to caring.

Surrounding the theoretical construct of the health-care relationship are multiple relationships and systems that reflect the lived reality of the patient and practitioner who function within relationships with family, community, organizations, and reimbursement structures. Although they may appear to be outside of the theoretical dyad, limitations and pressures such as financial reimbursement or health insurance can restrict the time a practitioner can spend with a patient and whether that consultation includes any time for patient education or counseling. Debates about health care contain implicit assumptions about the nature and the importance of the health-care relationship, and each profession will likely attempt to protect its unique understanding of that relationship.

Clinical practice guidelines are continually being developed from research and clinical evidence in an attempt to improve and standardize medical care. As algorithms are applied to patient groups or diagnoses, part of that calculation relies on the construct of an ideal patient who is willing and able to follow a regimen. Practical reality is often more complex. Patients bring to the health-care relationship a varied sense of agency and trust formed during prior experiences with authorities or professionals. A prolonged experience of feeling disenfranchised can create obstacles for participating in programs and regimens that are pre-

4. Meleis, *Theoretical Nursing.*
5. Delougery, *Issues and Trends in Nursing.*

sented as "being good for you." Resistance to professional advice is not limited to individuals and individual memories; the history of experimentation with targeted racial groups, such as in the Tuskegee Syphilis Study, leaves a persistent legacy of distrust in clinical trials.

Capacity on the part of the client refers to the willingness or ability to understand and retain information in order to arrive at a decision. Decision making in health care assumes an active agent, and part of the work of the health-care relationship is depicted as empowering this active agent to make responsible choices that lead to health or wellness. However, as Howard Thurman observes, the disinherited—those with their backs against the wall—live with a different sense of agency shaped by a fear that is a kind of death in itself.[6] The imposition of best practices and the dissemination of research into clinical guidelines rarely accounts for this variation in the patient side of the equation.

The treatment regimen may be doomed before it has begun. The client may be predisposed to ignore advice from educated professionals who presume to know what she needs. Beliefs shaped by class, ethnicity, religion, urban or rural location and relocation, as well as prior experience in the health-care system, can create complex patterns of client participation in the health-care relationship. How can the health-care practitioner be best prepared for the complexity and individual variation of a practitioner-client relationship?

The health-care relationship may be a onetime encounter or it can develop over time as in, for example, the case of chronic illness or cancer survivorship. Although the dyad appears to be a static entity, in reality the health-care relationship, like any other relationship, may cycle through points of frustration and anger, or experience cycles of optimism and disappointment. The practitioner in a long-term health-care relationship may also experience different emotions and frustrations over time working with a client or group of clients. Finally, the complexity of modern health care means that patients are treated by groups of professionals who change regularly, leaving the patient to begin a new health-care relationship with every encounter (with resulting duplication and re-telling of illness narratives).

Clients' religious and spiritual values can change over time, as their faith either grows through adversity or collapses under the burden of illness. Rather than being simply a private aspect of the individual's cul-

6. Thurman, *Jesus and the Disinherited*, 11.

ture with little relevance to the health-care relationship, spirituality can support the health-care relationship or undermine the work of the professional. The health-care relationship can be an important part in the spiritual shift and change that may accompany the illness experience.

Shame, stigma, or embarrassment rooted in religious beliefs can accompany and complicate the health-care relationship. Such beliefs may impede a client from following clinical advice or participating with mutuality in the health-care relationship. Although the role of resilience is still being debated in many fields, including psychology, one might assume that the client's spiritual or religious framework plays a role in that resilience or flourishing. Subtle or even unacknowledged judgment or criticism, or any difference in religious, class, or ethnic perspectives on the part of the practitioner may inhibit aspects of the health-care relationship.

SEEKING HELP

The client makes an appointment with a professional (or ends up in the emergency room) to seek help, advice, treatment, or a solution to a problem (or to be treated against her will). Help-seeking behavior includes the formal and informal supports provided by family, friends, traditional healers, and religious leaders.[7] The client may be assigned to a specific professional or group of professionals by insurance or geographic restrictions, or may seek someone whose credentials and experience match his or her need. The search for help may begin late in the experience of symptoms or at the beginning of onset. Ultimately the efficacy of treatment may depend on the timing of the search. For hospice care, for example, clients who are actively dying or in the end stages provide little opportunity for the staff to provide the full range of support services for the patient and family or to develop helping relationships with them.

EMPATHY AND THE HEALTH-CARE RELATIONSHIP

More and Milligan observe that the health-care relationship has been governed by norms that range from a detached practitioner to a more sympathetic and engaged interaction. Being sympathetic can be interpreted as undermining one's scientific credentials.[8] This notion of

7. Barker, *Adolescents, Social Support and Help-Seeking Behaviour.*

8. More and Milligan, eds., *Empathic Practitioner,* 23.

sympathy as a detrimental aspect arose in modern times; by contrast, Hippocratic practitioners were expected to have passion for their patients. Before doctors believed that detachment was a necessary part of the relationship, physicians in the time of Hippocrates were urged to eliminate selfish and destructive emotions to allow them to develop a special *philia*, an emotional experience, through which physicians are moved by the sufferings of patients.

James Hardee argues that empathy is a higher order of human relationship and understanding that he calls "engaged detachment." Sympathy steps into the suffering self, but empathy relies on "borrowing" so that we can observe, feel, and understand the other's feelings without taking them on.[9]

The root of therapeutic empathy is the ability of the physician to understand a patient's emotional point of view. Halpern believes that in the interpersonal realm, emotions are crucial for understanding reality, requiring physicians to practice reflection rather than detaching from emotions. This awareness will allow doctors to take better histories and to engage in more effective communication. Detachment does not make medicine more rational; it creates situations where emotions can go underground and give rise to irrational behaviors or cognitive distortions.[10] A lack of reflection on the daily realities of suffering can lead professionals to find solace in a variety of behaviors and distractions, none of which will ultimately provide comfort to the suffering self.

The attribution of innate abilities to empathize has often been ascribed to a particular gender or to a particular profession. When associated with the emotions, empathy was considered unreliable, unscientific, and unmanly. More notes that when psychoanalysis revalued empathy in the 1960s, the scientific character of empathy allowed it to be distanced from feminine characteristics and to be described as a technical instrument.[11] Professional training, as we have seen in chapter 1, stresses the unique and specialized knowledge of the professional. For many professionals, the ideal of empathy both characterizes the distinct claims of the professional and limits the scientific credibility of that profession. The tension between caring and competence means that professions either

9. Hardee, "Overview of Empathy."

10. Halpern, *From Detached Concern*, 17.

11. More and Milligan, eds., *Empathic Practitioner*, 23–29.

distance themselves from the notion of empathy or embrace it as defining what they do in relation to cultural and societal values of empathy.

RESPONSE TO THE ENCOUNTER— ADHERENCE AND COMPLIANCE

In the medical literature, the relationship between patient and practitioner has been constructed in ways that focus on the capacities of the doctor or on the failings of the patient. The notion of the dyad is a useful conceptual device to isolate key variables in this inquiry. In practice, however, neither the focus on a specific disease (for example, diabetes) or on a specific variable (for example, patient unwillingness or lack of understanding of drug regimen) are a true representation of the complexity of the encounter.

Theoretical understanding of the patient's response to treatment has been studied from the perspective of compliance or adherence. The construction of categories of patient behavior has at times resorted to interpreting patient's uncooperation as "deviance."[12] The very notion of patient response to advice assumes a professional who not only has authority based on specialized knowledge, but who also knows better than the patient what might be required.

Compliance first emerged in the literature on the patient-practitioner relationship in the 1950s. In the 1970s, the notion of compliance grew with Sackett and Haynes's work.[13] The wave of compliance research in this decade coincided with the increasing number of pharmaceuticals available—a possibility that required physicians to understand patient cooperation in drug treatment regimens. The investigations focused on questions such as: How many patients do not take treatments as instructed, What are the characteristics of these patients, and Why did they not follow instructions? Empathy was not necessarily part of the concern with patient behavior; the efficacy of drugs and the potential profits of pharmaceutical breakthroughs were essential.

In a study of themes in the compliance literature, Lutfey and Wishner identified shifts in research questions from demographic characteristics of patients to psychological characteristics and larger social issues, such as patients' beliefs about their health regimens, as well as

---

12. Lerner, "Careless Consumptives to Recalcitrant Patients," 1423–31.
13. Haynes et al., *Compliance in Health Care.*

social and economic resources that help people seek and follow medical advice. Studies focused on communication skills of the practitioner or attachment styles of the patient. Those with secure attachment styles demonstrated better health outcomes, whereas patients with dismissing attachment style had poorer health outcomes.[14]

The term "adherence" has largely replaced the older term "compliance," which was associated with a dominance model of medical practice wherein the patient was expected to be obedient and follow all recommendations in a passive way. In the context of the psychiatric survivor movement, such imposition of regimens on patients became suspect. Traditionally the term "compliance" reflected a patient's response to prescribed treatment. General theories of compliance literature include the following: compliance to medication;[15] mental health compliance;[16] and compliance in specific conditions, such as asthma or hypertension.[17]

Compliance is discussed from the perspective of patient education,[18] diet,[19] and screening.[20] Increasingly, however, the term raises questions for researchers about the assumptions related to the medical model of compliance[21] and the ethics of compliance.[22] Narrow studies on patient behavior and compliance are increasingly criticized as missing the full reality of the context and setting within which the health-care relationship evolves.

Although there is general agreement that a health-care relationship exists whenever a patient/client and practitioner meet to discuss the patient's care, there are diverse views about the nature of that relationship and its effect on outcomes. Adherence has been proposed as an alternate way to understand the health-care relationship. In contrast to the concept of compliance, which sees the patient within a paternalistic system and labels behavior as not in accord with the directions given, the concept of adherence is based on a health-care relationship, wherein

14. Thompson and Ciechanowski, "Attaching a New Understanding," 419–26.

15. Salzman, "Medication Compliance," 18–22.

16. Bhui, "Language of Compliance," 157–63.

17. Chapman et al., "Improving Patient Compliance," 2–9.

18.. Brus et al., "Compliance in Rheumatoid Arthritis," 702–10.

19.. Luft et al., "Compliance to a Low-Salt Diet," 698S–703S.

20. Neilson and Whynes, "Determinants of Persistent Compliance," 365–74.

21. Ward-Collins, "Noncompliant," 27–31.

22. Hess, "Ethics of Compliance," 18–27.

power is shared with the professional. Within this re-visioned relationship, mutual respect sets the tone of the encounter that results in enhanced health-care outcomes. Adherence has been defined as the extent to which a patient's behavior is consistent with the health-care provider's recommendations (World Health Organization, 2003). Adherence to recommended treatment regimen in the pediatric population for all conditions ranges from 43 percent to 100 percent, with just half of children, on average, adhering to recommended treatment.[23] Although many factors have been investigated with both adults and children for their association with nonadherence to recommended treatment, none have consistently shown to be significant predictors.[24]

Studies of adherence and relational factors of care are studied in the context of specific diseases, medication adherence, the role of communication factors, and the role of patient communication—the literature in this area continues to grow. Spirituality and religiosity have also been studied in relation to adherence. In a study of patients with congestive heart failure, researchers found that religious commitment was the sole predictor of adherence to CHF-related behaviors, an effect that remained when controlling for initial levels of adherence.[25] Spirituality and religious factors can also affect adherence negatively when stigma complicates health-seeking behavior. Individual beliefs and the health encounter can affect each other in positive or negative ways.

A study of rates of adherence with HIV regimens indicated that religious beliefs could play a negative role in treatment adherence due to the stigma attached to HIV disease, particularly in geographical areas and in population subgroups where religious practices are strong. In this exploratory study, HIV-positive individuals in a southern state were surveyed as to their attitudes and beliefs surrounding HIV disease and adherence to medical treatment for the disease.[26] The results indicated that multiple factors influence adherence to treatment and that certain religious practices are positively associated with adherence, but certain religious beliefs can be negatively related to adherence. Spirituality, religiosity, faith, and cultural background are complex factors in health-care behavior and in the health-care relationship, and these are factors

23. Burkhart and Rayens, "Self Concept and Health Locus of Control," 404–10.

24. Park et al., "Religiousness and Treatment Adherence," 249–66.

25. Ibid.

26. Parsons et al., "Religious Beliefs, Practices, and Treatment Adherence," 97–111.

for which researchers, clinicians, and professional students receive little training.

Adherence is rarely 100 percent with any treatment—rates have reportedly ranged from 25 to 95 percent.[27] Empathy seems to have some role in this response to treatment; the rate of following advice tends to increase with increased empathy shown by the practitioner, including communication style and willingness to answer patient questions.[28] Adherence, the literature suggests, allows relational factors of care to be linked to health outcomes. Despite the difficulties involved in quantifying the role of empathy in health outcomes, it has been argued that a positive patient-practitioner relationship can lead to the following positive outcomes: patient satisfaction with health care and with the practitioner, diagnostic accuracy, better engagement with the therapeutic regimen, and shorter length of hospitalizations.

Studies of adherence are often one-sided, scrutinizing patient behavior rather than studying the mutuality of the health-care relationship. To fully capture the reality of the interaction, research needs to include the health-care relationship, adherence, and changes in disease severity as well.[29]

Considering the difficulties of quantifying the effects of the heathcare relationship, or more specifically of empathy, can one assume that there are mutual benefits of the health-care relationship? Among the benefits that patients derive from the relationship, Hojat includes adherence to treatment regimens; satisfaction with the health-care provider and the health-care system; recall and understanding of medical information; ability to cope with the disease; improvement in the quality of life; and physical, mental, and social well-being. A large body of literature supports the notion that the physician-patient relationship can facilitate the process of patient care and have a positive effect on health outcomes. Hojat observes that of twenty-one published studies, sixteen reported a statistically significant positive correlation between effective positive patient-physician relationships and effective outcomes.[30]

27. Eisenthal et al., "'Adherence' and the Negotiated Approach to Parenthood," 393–98.

28. Hojat, *Empathy in Patient Care*, 169.

29. Di Matteo et al., "Health Beliefs," 521–28.

30. Hojat, *Empathy in Patient Care*, 119.

However, the benefits of this relationship and the empathy that makes it possible are not limited to the client alone. Hojat notes the benefits of empathy for the clinician: "The good news is that clinicians' satisfaction with their relationships with patients can serve as a buffer against the professional stress, burnout, substance abuse, and even suicide attempts that are reported to be unusually high among health professionals."[31] Empathy thus emerges as an important factor, not only in patient behavior and health outcomes, but also in the experience of the practitioner in ensuring satisfaction with one's career.

ISOLATING THE RELATIONAL FACTORS IN THE HEALTH-CARE RELATIONSHIP

Empathy can form the basis for active listening and openness to the reality of the other. Connelly notes that problems may arise when the physician does not make listening a priority: "Understanding does not occur, empathy is compromised, the therapeutic alliance may not develop, healing is minimized, and suffering may result."[32] Empathy can never replace technical excellence on the part of the practitioner. One eye must always be focused on the procedure, the regimen, the surgery, the treatment; the other eye can focus on the relational aspects of care.

If empathy is allowed into the relationship, it is easier to see that the health-care relationship can be a relational co-creation. Instead of viewing the patient side of the relationship as a variable to be controlled or manipulated through communication or other techniques, one might imagine the patient response as active co-creation, in which silence, conflict, nonacceptance, anger or nonadherence are not failures, but form significant relational aspects of the health-care relationship.

If one assumes that empathy is the factor that makes relational care and mutuality possible, what are the components of empathy and the associated competencies that professionals need to develop? Some of these might include active listening, nonjudgmental presence, self-disclosure, healthy professional boundaries, and an ability to engage in reflection. Empathy is described here as an overall category that includes a variety of skills and attitudes that can enhance the relationship. Improving professional communication skills are only one part of these relational

31. Ibid.
32. Connelly, "Empathic Practitioner: Empathy, Gender, and Medicine," 171–88.

skills, but studies have shown that training can improve skills and confidence as part of relational abilities.[33] If professional educators believe that empathy can make a difference in the outcomes of encounters, such as through the health-care relationship, the definition of the requisite skills, knowledge, and attitudes will be an essential part of curriculum development and assessment.

EFFECTS OF EMPATHY IN THE PATIENT-PRACTITIONER RELATIONSHIP

No one definition is sufficient in considering the meaning of empathy. Indeed, empathy is often considered an elusive concept that is sufficiently complex to increase the diversity of its meaning.[34] Empathy, according to Bennett, involves a mode of relating "in which one person comes to know the mental content of another, both affectively and cognitively, at a particular moment in time and as a product of the relationship that exists between them."[35] Hojat indicates that empathy is an elusive concept full of conceptual ambiguity, but despite this ambiguity "empathy is among the most frequently mentioned humanistic dimensions of patient care."[36]

These attempts at definition reveal an underlying complexity in the concept. This complexity increases as one attempts to apply empathy to the patient-practitioner relationship. For the psychotherapeutic encounter, empathy is what builds the nonjudgmental or unconditional positive regard of the therapist. Such acceptance opens up self-acceptance or a more accurately based self for the client.[37]

On the relationship between choice and control, Candib argues that "mutual recognition of the patient's needs (dependency) can be viewed as empowering for the patient" if the practitioner pays attention to the client and through active listening attempts to see how the patient can be helped to make choices that are empowering.[38] In practice, then, this understanding of empathy means that the clinician enters the patient's

---

33. Meyer et al., "Difficult Conversations," 352–59.
34. Feshbach, "Empathy," 35–39.
35. Bennett, ed., *Empathic Healer*, 7.
36. Hojat, *Empathy in Patient Care*, 7.
37. Bozarth, "Empathy from the Framework of Client-Centered Theory," 85.
38. Candib, "Reconsidering Power," 135–56.

world and attempts to understand it, allowing both to be affected by the experience. Part of this work involves paying attention to the patient's story and using responsible disclosure to develop mutuality. Research on this relationship cannot rely on an objective interviewer but must include personal involvement between the researcher and the interviewee and the sharing of information in a way that empowers the patient.

Although empathy may have a bearing on outcomes, the difficulty of defining empathy creates problems for researchers. These definitional issues impede the study of positive outcomes tied to the relational aspects of care, including greater patient satisfaction or reduced litigation. How can engagement in empathic understanding also change the experience or the encounter for the practitioner, allowing for increased satisfaction, lower burnout or job stress, and better health outcomes? An empathic encounter would require a holistic and engaged approach characterized by a mutuality of interest and power. The admission of uncertainty and the sharing of vulnerability appear to contradict the ideology of a profession that relies on expertise and control. In a professional setting, can a student learn or be mentored to participate in this kind of mutuality?

Three skills associated with empathy in clinical situations are the abilities to identify emotions in oneself and others, to assume the perspective of others, and to express emotion in a controlled, articulate manner.[39] That such skills are valued in different professions is evident in their practice guidelines; the ability to establish a therapeutic relationship is regarded as an essential skill. Empathy is named as one of the requisite capacities for establishing therapeutic relationships. The American Association of Medical Colleges underscores empathy as an essential learning objective because empathy is believed to significantly influence patient satisfaction, adherence to medical recommendations, clinical outcomes, and professional satisfaction.[40]

MEASUREMENT OF EMPATHY

Scales and tests have been devised to help ascertain whether one has empathy. Empathy is increasingly studied from within psychology and biology in an attempt to provide more quantitative measures. Studies on

---

39. Feshbach, "Empathy," 52.
40. Stepien and Baernstein, "Educating for Empathy."

empathy include the effects of empathic failure by a parent, which results in a child who is unable to have perspective or critically reflect.

People who have suffered empathic failure from parents will have trouble processing their own experiences; that, in turn, might compromise their ability to moderate the intensity of an experience or to attend to the experience of another person without losing the ability to return to their own experience. Clients who have a fragile style of processing tend to experience core issues at very high or low levels of intensity and have difficultly stopping or starting experiences that are personally significant or emotionally connected. In addition, they are likely to have difficulty taking the point of view of another person while remaining in contact with their own experiences.[41]

In order to quantify measures of improvement in patient adherence, the need for scales or measures of such effects are increasingly valued. Admissions tests for professional schools may eventually consider screening applicants on the basis of noncognitive personality traits rather than cognitive tests, which have been criticized for putting certain groups at a disadvantage.[42] Admission tests, such as the Multiple Mini Interview (MMI), are now being used by twelve of Canada's seventeen medical schools, as well as by schools of dentistry, nursing, and midwifery. In an article in the *Globe and Mail* (18 May 2009), McMaster University professor Dr. Rosenfeld states, "We recognized that our biggest problem is not in evaluating the cognitive domain—it's not about knowledge. It's the interpersonal domain: the way of dealing with people. It's about ethics and it's about judgment." Identifying the capacity in applicants and tying that capacity to educational intervention will remain a challenge for professional schools.

SPIRITUALITY

If empathy could be considered a stance towards the world that leads to a way of engaging in the world and working towards a common good, how would one name or locate this capacity? Could the notion of empathy find a place in the world of empirical and quantifiable reality? Philosopher Martin Buber refers to an inherent relationality that is prior to any action and greater than any sentiment. In this relational existence,

41. Warner, "Does Empathy Cure?" 125–40.
42. Chen, "Do You Have the Right Stuff?"

"Our students teach us, our works inform us."[43] Such relationality can be considered part of the realm of the spiritual nature of existence. According to Miller, a spiritual perspective means that "we see ourselves connected to something larger than ourselves."[44] One aspect of learning from a spiritual perspective, according to Miller, requires compassionate knowing—a recognition that we are part of an interconnected universe. Teachers need compassion to see themselves in their students, and students feel safe in the presence of a compassionate teacher. Increased attention in health care to the importance of spiritual care for patients has created new opportunities for defining the role and importance of spirituality. Recognizing that spiritual care is an important part of the patient's context and culture with significant effects on health-care outcomes marks an important cultural and educational shift in professional education and culture.

Hospitals are providing multifaith chaplaincies and interdisciplinary initiatives to improve the effectiveness of their interventions. With that increased attention, new standards and guidelines for quality spiritual care are being developed. Puchalski describes the work of a Consensus Conference in California in 2009 to create guidelines for quality spiritual care.[45] Innovations, organizational recognitions of the importance of a spiritual realm or a relational priority, and new research findings and creative programming will continue to explore relationality and its role in the health-care relationship. Empathy may emerge in this professional relationship as an essential element to the professional relationship and one that provides positive outcomes for both clients and professionals. This may require a shift in recognition of different ways of knowing and experiencing. In the next chapter, we will look at how professionals are taught to regard (or ignore) suffering and how that regard is an essential step in the ability to extend empathy.

---

43. Buber, *I and Thou*, 67.

44. Miller, "Learning from a Spiritual Perspective," 95–102.

45. Puchalski et al., "Improving the Quality of Spiritual Care," 885–904.

QUESTIONS FOR FURTHER DISCUSSION

1. Do you recall an incident when someone extended empathy to you? Describe that incident and your feelings at the time.

2. What is the difference between adherence and compliance? Search online for recent articles that use this language.

3. What language is used to describe a client's response to advice in other professional relationships such as teaching or social work? What does that language suggest about the relationship between the professional and the client?

4. In your profession, what types of models of the professional relationship are used to describe the client-professional interaction? Have these changed over time? How?

5. Research one of the scales or measures of empathy. What are the strengths and weaknesses of this type of measurement tool?

6. How does your profession support the diversity of beliefs and background of clients? Do you use an interviewing tool that captures the spiritual history of a client? If not, can you imagine designing such a tool?

7. Describe what you feel are the characteristics of a therapeutic relationship.

PART TWO

Learning Empathic Engagement

3

Regarding Suffering

MY FRIEND JANE WAS admitted to the emergency room of a busy urban hospital after having a seizure at home. While talking to her on the phone, I heard the phone fall from her hand while she had what was later determined to be a grand mal seizure. Another friend had been having tea with her, so she had called the ambulance that took Jane to the university hospital. I raced downtown to the urban hospital when I got her message. I was not allowed immediate access to Jane because tests were being done. Locating a hard plastic chair in the waiting room, I tried to tune out the relentless noise of the TV and the ugliness of the florescent-lit waiting room. I wished I had brought something to read.

Two young children slept in one corner, leaning against each other, with no parent in sight. Another woman moaned in pain as her grand-daughter tried to comfort her. The security guard blocked the door to the patient care area and ignored those in the waiting area while a triage nurse interviewed the next patient in line. The entire setting created an inhospitable space.

When I was finally allowed to enter the curtained cubicle where Jane was trying to deal with a severe headache, the nurse placed EKG chest leads on her while ignoring both of us. She pulled the patient gown up to Jane's neck without a warning and exposed her breasts with no concern for her modesty. Jane was clearly embarrassed by the lack of privacy. Only an hour before, she had been an independent person—a professional, with a career and friends. Within moments of arriving at the hospital, Jane was given a new identity based on illness. Her choices were either to resist or submit.

Through the curtain, the nurse carried on a conversation with a coworker about how inebriated she had been at a party the previous night. I realized that the nurse was functioning in an automatic way that was technically correct, but she missed an opportunity to connect with the patient. I was tempted to point out this behavior to the nurse, but kept silent because I knew that my friend would pay in numerous ways if we irritated her nurse. Being labeled a problem or difficult patient would not be helpful for my friend.

Practitioners who receive clients into the care of an organization or clinic provide the first point of contact for the patient. Consider the following questions:

1. What might the nurse have done differently in this situation?

2. What messages was the nurse giving the patient about her body and about her illness?

3. If you were the patient, how would you feel in this situation?

4. What kinds of suffering were happening here? As a helping professional, what would be your role in this situation?

5. Write your own definition of suffering.

6. What are the policy implications of the use of urgent care in your location?

DEFINING THE PERSON

The notion of suffering is sometimes lost in the focus on specific aspects of treatment regimens, outcomes, learning goals, quality improvement, and sheer overwork. In health care, the suffering of the patient and family are traditionally the responsibility of the nurses and pastoral staff who have more intimate and daily knowledge of the patient's situation. In some settings such as palliative and hospice care, interdisciplinary conferences bring staff together to talk about the overall situation of the patient and to compare perspectives. The notion of entering imaginatively into each other's practices counters decades of specialization and parallel practice, as well as the professionalizing strategy that seeks to contain expertise and protect boundaries.

Professional training often has little room for suffering as a guiding concept for care. The notion of suffering disrupts Western beliefs in progress and technological advances that promise to cure or at least extend life. Suffering also carries connotations of religious and philosophical inquiries that seem more suited to the humanities than to the work of science.

Advances in medicine have indeed brought cures and extended life expectancy, but survivors of cancer and other diseases or those with chronic illnesses experience altered lives under conditions that may include suffering. For those in the helping professions, suffering in all its forms will be their daily focus. As medicine has increasingly specialized, the body has been divided up according to professional expertise. In a postmodern culture, what does it mean to suffer? And who is there to witness that suffering? How can students be prepared to recognize the many forms that suffering can take? And can they be taught to reflect on their own suffering as they encounter the myriad ways that children, young adults, and adults suffer?

Even though the obligation for physicians to relieve human suffering goes back to antiquity, Eric Cassell observes that little attention is given to the subject in medical education, research, or practice. In order for medicine to understand what suffering is and how physicians might be devoted to its relief, medicine must overcome "its traditional dichotomy between mind and body, subjective and objective, and person and object." [1] When personhood is restricted to mind, spirit, and the subject, the notion of suffering becomes a private matter of that domain. Suffering, he argues, occurs when "an impending destruction of the person is perceived; it continues until the threat of disintegration has passed or until the integrity of the person can be restored in some other manner."[2] Under the rubric of personhood, Cassell includes all the components of an individual's complexity, such as family, life experiences, cultural background, roles, and relationships, as well as a transcendent dimension. Such multifaceted creatures cannot be reduced to mechanical injury but have a potential for injury and suffering that is complex.

THE BIOMEDICAL SYSTEM AND (DIS)REGARD OF SUFFERING

Recent scholarship recognizes that biomedicine has supported crucial innovations in medicine but also shapes the culture in which practitioners deal with patients. Medical anthropologist Arthur Kleinman observes that biomedicine reduces life to nature as a physical and knowable

---

1. Cassell, *Nature of Suffering*, 32.
2. Ibid.

object.[3] Biomedicine, according to anthropologist Margaret Lock, is a product of the nineteenth-century emergence of biology, where nature is understood as comprised of laws independent of both society and culture. The shift meant that disease and health could be "assessed and controlled independent of the circumstances in which individuals are situated."[4]

For practitioners of biomedicine, the focus is on constructing disease using objective data while disregarding the patient's subjective experience of suffering. Although not opposed to progress in biomedicine, Kleinman laments the loss of "a humanly significant relationship of witnessing, affirming, and engaging the patient and family's existential experience."[5] By denying the patient and family experience, and possibly pastoral care givers as well, doctors in effect deny patients and their families and other helping professions an opportunity to pass through suffering and to make sense of the ultimate meaning of life. Biomedicine decontextualizes diagnostics and therapeutics to the interior of the body or to individual behavior, and ultimately it is removed from the moral realm. The notion that biomedicine is free of "cultural and moral evaluation is itself a moral position."[6]

As biomedicine grew into an increasingly bureaucratized and rationalized system, the health care division of labor became divided into systems: diagnosis and prescription to doctors; care of the body to nurses; and spirituality increasingly to professionalized clergy. One disadvantage of this rationalized system was that each of these care groups was shaped by the culture of their professional education (whether based primarily in the humanities or in science), and there were few opportunities to share observations or to gain insight from shared knowledge. The fracture of science from humanities has been further consolidated by the postmodern insistence on the relative and private nature of each individual's beliefs. Some communities see their own strengths in contrast to biomedicine and refuse to submit to the reductionism involved in modern medicine. In a study of African-American healing, Stephanie Mitchem notes that concepts of the body and healing in black culture contrast sharply with those of institutional

3. Kleinman, *Writing at the Margin*.
4. Lock, "Medical Knowledge and Body Politics," 192.
5. Kleinman, *Writing at the Margin*, 21–37.
6. Lock, "Medical Knowledge and Body Politics," 196.

medicine. Relationships are central to healing processes and acts in which the body has meaning because of connections with "the past, the future, the family, and the divine."[7]

INDIVIDUAL SUFFERING

Suffering is a universal human experience located in the body, mind, spirit, or in a combination of those aspects. Rather than isolating suffering in one aspect, one can regard the person as a whole; thus, when health is diminished in one aspect of human life, other areas are also affected.[8] Although some individuals do not encounter suffering until they are mature adults, others experience it already from birth or at a very young age. Halpern notes that in suffering, "expectations about the reliability of the world and of one's capacity to achieve any of one's goals can be destroyed."[9] Thus, suffering has the potential to provoke a crisis of faith, not necessarily in the sense of religion, but in one's view of the world and one's place in it. Suffering also has the capacity to build new capacities for care, gratitude, and appreciation for life.

Suffering is an interruption to one's sense of the world that challenges presuppositions about one's identity, purpose, and expectations of how the future would unfold. Suffering can provoke a transformative experience similar to the process that Jack Mezirow describes for adult learning, wherein education causes a shift in frames of reference and a restructuring of frames to incorporate new knowledge.[10] Suffering can provide a disorienting dilemma that results in a rethinking of previously held assumptions. Suffering individuals sometimes describe their experience as transformative—a language that is shared by adult educators. That is not to suggest that individuals should seek out suffering in order to be transformed. The health care practitioner can, however, be influential in helping an individual seek wholeness in the face of changes that are potentially transformative, even when the individual can never return to the state of being experienced prior to illness. The new frame of reference may include a new way of inhabiting the body or of experiencing the world.

---

7. Mitchem and Townes, "Faith, Health, and Healing," 186.

8. Doornbos et al., *Transforming Care*, 78.

9. Halpern, *From Detached Concern*, 112.

10. Mezirow, *Transformative Dimensions*.

An important part of this re-sorting of values and meaning is the opportunity to lament what has been lost. Nursing professor Mary Doornbos distinguishes lament from despair and argues that nurses work with the double vision of shalom that "allows us to see what is not yet, while at the same time we see what we are called to at this time."[11] Lament is an essential part of both individual and communal experience of suffering as well as the movement towards healing. Although suffering is often described for the individual, it is important that helping professionals recognize how suffering is shared and experienced communally through such practices as lament and ritual. Lament as such enables the expression and sharing of suffering and the questioning of larger issues of justice.[12] For helping professionals, a willingness to face the suffering other and to transcend a particular belief system in order to understand each patient is a challenge that properly begins in professional school and continues throughout one's career. An appreciation of the intercultural and interreligious ways that communities and individuals experience and express suffering is an essential skill that can allow the professional to engage with the client and family in meaningful ways. In addition, such an ability to engage with the suffering other demands an awareness of the suffering self.

SOURCES OF SUFFERING & THE SUFFERER EXPERIENCE

The source of suffering may be a physical condition present at birth, such as a congenital anomaly; a physical condition acquired through illness or injury; an emotional state or mental illness; or a combination of these. Some children grow up in conditions that do not allow them to thrive because they lack physical or emotional basics or because they have been subjected to emotional or physical abuse. Essential for all helping professions is a critical awareness of the systemic causes of suffering.

When suffering is a result of illness or disease, theories of natural causation (infection, stress, organic deterioration, accident, or overt human aggression) may be used as an explanation. Many cultures rely on theories of supernatural causation to explain disease and illness, including mystical causation, animistic causation, and magical causation. The experience of suffering is expressed through metaphors and culturally

---

11. Doornbos et al., *Transforming Care*, 77.

12. Mitchem and Townes, "Faith, Health, and Healing," 87–89.

constructed narratives that help the individual and the family or community deal with feelings and anxiety about the experience.[13]

PAIN

Pain can accompany suffering, but pain is not essential to defining what constitutes a suffering experience. Because pain tolerance differs greatly between individuals, an injury that might be experienced as a mere nuisance to one person might be devastating to another. Some individuals might faint at the sight of an injury, whereas others would not require anesthetic for some procedures. Each individual situation alters the experience of suffering; for example, a foot injury would be experienced differently by someone whose mobility was essential to his or her job, compared to someone who could work at a computer. Some individuals withdraw when faced with suffering; others seek community to survive the experience. Each person thus experiences suffering differently, and no system can predict the individual response to suffering.

The professional who regards and evaluates suffering will be influenced by his or her own notion of suffering. How we answer the *why* of suffering can affect how we experience or endure it, and how we regard the suffering of another. Diana Cates distinguishes emotional pain from physical pain. Physical pain takes as its object a particular bodily sensation, and emotional pain takes as its object some occurrence or circumstance in the larger world of personal experience.[14] Part of suffering is related to our intactness as persons and the sense of loss "in relation to the world of objects, events and relationships," sustaining a sense of loss that comes not just from the body, but from the web of relationships that surrounds a person.[15] Supporting the loss, grief, altered identity, changed relations, and uncertainty that illness brings is a challenge for all levels of helping professions. It also offers the potential for deep engagement in the suffering of another.

ISOLATION

Suffering can either isolate the individual from normal life or can ultimately bind that person into communion with others. The experience

13. Singer and Baer, *Introducing Medical Anthropology*, 70.
14. Cates, *Choosing to Feel*, 139.
15. Cassell, *Nature of Suffering*, 40.

of suffering may ultimately increase the individual's ability to identify with others who suffer. The exact mechanics of this increased sensitivity to suffering is unclear; perhaps as the more social and inauthentic self is dismantled by suffering, the senses are more open to hearing the pain of others. While sharing the pain of another, we generally do not experience the exact same sensation; however, Cates argues it is possible to share a similar set of experiences.[16] Those who have a very high capacity for empathy might in fact be quite vulnerable to developing similar symptoms as the client with whom they are identifying—and for those students, training is necessary to manage this wealth of empathic feeling that might threaten their own health.

TIME

Time is a factor in suffering, because suffering depends on whether the condition causing it is acute and treatable or chronic and ongoing. To the person who is suffering, the perception of time can be distorted as suffering takes them into a realm of experience disconnected from daily routines. Cassell notes that suffering will influence people's perception of the future; if pain is perceived as taking over the future, people fear they will be overwhelmed.[17] David Kahn and Richard Steeves note that suffering disrupts not only the sense of time, but also people's sense of embodiment and the social world, in the form of human relationships.[18] Certain forms of suffering distort time to such an extent that the future can no longer be visualized, as in the case of trauma.

CUMULATIVE SUFFERING

Suffering can be cumulative. For example, Diane spent two hours at the dentist undergoing a root canal procedure. Then, because her appointment had already been set, she also underwent a routine cleaning. During the second procedure, she was so uncomfortable that she burst into tears and asked the hygienist to stop. The cumulative effect of the discomfort reached a point where she could no longer bear it. As a practitioner, it is difficult to see the cumulative suffering that a client has endured over time because the practitioner is often focusing on a discrete presenting

16. Cates, *Choosing to Feel*, 140.

17. Cassell, *Nature of Suffering*, 36.

18. Kahn and Steeves, "Understanding of Suffering," 3–28.

event. The history is an important part of the client narrative, not only for diagnostic information, but also for a more complete understanding of the experience of illness over time.

Suffering can be so intense that the individual person feels obliterated. French philosopher Simone Weil (1909–1943) describes this immense suffering as affliction. Weil notes that there are three types of affliction: physical pain, social exclusion, and spiritual distress. Weil believed that in the deepest affliction one could be attuned to the truth of God.[19]

Theologian Dorothee Soelle affirms the view that some suffering goes beyond pain and affects every dimension of life, to the point that "no discourse is possible any longer, in which a person ceases reacting as a human agent."[20] The dehumanizing effects of affliction or intense suffering impede human action and leave clients unable to act or speak.

THE BODY

Suffering may begin in one domain, such as the body, and may precipitate or be joined by suffering in another. For example, one student finishing a residency in dental surgery developed a condition where she could not use her arm. When the condition appeared to be permanent, the student grieved the loss of her chosen profession and became depressed. Bodily suffering resulted in a suffering spirit. The doctor who treated her was primarily concerned with healing her arm, a healing that did not seem to be forthcoming. After several months of depression, the woman consulted a counselor who facilitated the verbalization of fears related to the loss of her chosen profession and the change in her identity. Prior to this physical setback, she had never questioned her own success or experienced any obstacles to obtaining her goals. She confessed that she had felt immune to such suffering, protected by her professional qualifications and her success. Her experience of suffering contained an intrapersonal element, wherein she worked to integrate new information about herself, and an interpersonal aspect, wherein professionals worked with her physical symptoms and her emotional experience of suffering.[21]

---

19. Weil, *Gravity and Grace.*

20. Soelle, *Suffering,* 68.

21. Kahn and Steeves, "Understanding of Suffering," 23.

It is important to note that such processes occur simultaneously while the patient is coping with the experience of suffering.

Suffering is experienced in and through the body, but that suffering is also interpreted through the lenses of gender, race, class, age, ethnicity, religious or spiritual perspectives, personal history, and context. Suffering interrupts the "normal" routines of daily life and exposes core beliefs for critical examination. That reassessment of the taken-for-granted nature of one's daily life (work, relationships) may also involve a deeper confrontation with values, such as the meaning of life and the transience of one's experience. Although such an encounter with either unexamined or deeply-held values through suffering may seem unavoidable, Western culture provides endless distractions from the task. Suffering might offer transformation; however, such an outcome is not inevitable since some may resist changes imposed by illness to previously held beliefs.

A practitioner will encounter a wide variety of beliefs related to suffering and disease causation that may differ tremendously from his or her own beliefs. The role of empathy in encountering suffering is to stand with the individual or community in the face of suffering, with willingness to imagine how things might feel for the other. Such "standing with" requires suspension of the tendency to judge or to criticize the other for beliefs that contradict one's own. A professional will allow clients to express their sadness through lament, to experience weakness, and to search for new perspectives through this experience.

HEALING PLACE

When hospice care was first established at St. Christopher's Hospice in England (1967) and at the Connecticut Hospice in the United States (1980), architecture was considered an essential part of the mission to provide end-of-life care. Unfortunately, the same priority for the environment of care is generally ignored in most hospitals and clinics.

After accompanying his young daughter through a medical crisis, designer John Thackara observed that because medical knowledge is embodied, the design of work environments needs to enhance tacit and embodied knowledge. He observed that ultimately the best exchange of information occurs in a collaborative situation, with face-to-face exchange. Some organizations have attempted to design space with natural light, a small garden, or a labyrinth to counter the often impersonal and desolate spaces where care is given.[22]

SOCIAL SUFFERING

Although many studies focus on the individual, suffering is also a social experience. The voicelessness of suffering creates further isolation and marginalization—loss of voice may ultimately result in a total shattering of self. Suffering is "a social status that we extend or withhold . . . depending largely on whether the sufferer falls within our moral community."[23] In the case of trauma, survivors and communities are not faced with a life/death opposition, but experience a living death in the midst of their survival.

In writing about holocaust survivors, Lawrence Langer distinguishes between chronological time and durational time. The testimony of survivors can sound chronological to the listener, but narrators also inhabit durational time that places them outside of ordinary time. Memories are not ordered sequentially into a pattern from which one can be liberated. Finding new ways of telling a story, attaining political power from the margins, establishing paths to healing that involve the rebirth of traditions all provide challenges to oppressed communities who have experienced oppression and suffering.

When communities experience harsh physical conditions, natural disasters, or forms of oppression such as institutional racism, economic inequity, genocide, or poverty, the resulting communal suffering denies them the opportunity to be fully human. Social suffering is a term used to link the individual experience of suffering to wider social events and structural conditions.

The intergenerational and enduring aspects of this suffering have not been sufficiently documented. In displacements, individuals and communities in transition through immigration or forced relocation suffer a variety of physical and emotional disorders. Recent research demonstrates that trauma can be inherited by subsequent generations. Cross-generational passage of trauma is a subject of growing scholarly interest to neurobiologists and psychologists. Donna Nagata examines the cross-generational impact of the Japanese American internment;

---

22. Thackara, *In the Bubble*, 110–11. See also Wright and Adams, *Sacred Space*.
23. Kleinman et al., *Social Suffering*, 58.

the Sansei Research project uses a cross-generational framework to examine the transmission of trauma and injustice from the Nisei to the Sansei generation. Among the many findings, Nagata observes that severe injustices produce effects that extend far beyond the individuals who experienced the unjust event. The internment reminds many Sansei that Japanese Americans suffered a grave wrong, and thus many feel responsible for preventing injustices in their own world.[24] Research continues to examine the resilience as well as the suffering of generations affected by trauma or violence; for example, the neurobiology of trauma and the use of pharmacological interventions is the focus of ongoing research.

Communal suffering is complex and overwhelming to the individual. When the complexity of the suffering has been misread and the cure addresses only one aspect but ignores another, such as providing education with no opportunities for jobs, the proposed solution may not take root or may be met with resistance. Communities that have lost their connection to their historic identity or their spiritual roots cannot be cured by mere physical interventions. Affliction can require a spiritual cure, as well as physical and practical interventions. A variety of aboriginal programs for youth and adults refer to the return to the sacred as an adoption of native practices that bring healing to individuals and to the earth.

What does a broken or suffering spirit look like in communities of oppression and suffering, and how is it expressed in health and illness? Suffering is evident in increased rates of mortality, traumatic injury or death, hospitalization for pneumonia, and adolescent suicide. Suffering is also expressed in the increased incidence of Type II diabetes, asthma, and heart disease in both aboriginal communities and African-American communities. How can a helping professional respond to the suffering of communities and the individuals within them whose suffering is shaped by structural inequalities? The first step is learning to regard the suffering without judgment and with close awareness of and reflection on any personal discomfort.

As an outsider to the suffering of a particular community, how can one ever understand the complexity of suffering in addition to the resistance that accompanies it? Medical anthropologist Nancy Scheper-Hughes returned to a field site in Brazil where she had worked years be-

24. Nagata, *Legacy of Injustice*, 215.

fore. During her early fieldwork in Brazil in the 1960s, Scheper-Hughes sought to keep a positive view of the shantytown by attributing the misery she witnessed to external causes such as poverty, racism, class exploitation, and imperialism. Her research was guided by an assumption that was common to Western scholars; she observed the people and projected her own assumptions of sameness onto them. She assumed that underneath cultural difference, human beings were essentially alike. These assumptions did not help her explain why women seemed to be indifferent to the deaths of their small children. She found that she and the people did not understand each other, and she was faced with the opacity of culture. Seeming maternal indifference in Brazil was matched by bureaucratic and church indifference, leaving the social determinants of child death hidden from view. What seemed like indifference on the part of the women was actually a deeper response to structural poverty and hopelessness.[25]

Scheper-Hughes attempted to articulate the suffering of both the women and children while being aware of the impossibility of finding speech for those too young to speak. Concerning this challenge, she realized that her options were limited to one stance, namely, that of "being there" and "bearing witness" to the suffering of the silent or silenced others—in this instance, mothers and babies. She begins with an assumption of difference and avoids "all 'essentializing' and 'universalizing' discourses, whether they originate in the biomedical and psychological sciences or in philosophical or cultural feminism."[26]

Regarding suffering can mean encountering an unexplored landscape of incomprehensible difference that challenges one's most basic and unexamined assumptions. For many professional students, the confrontation with otherness can generate deep discomfort, anxiety, anger, and a desire to turn away. Despite the recognition of deep difference, one must sometimes struggle to find that which binds people in common human relation, even when no connection can be imagined. A clinician interprets the behavior of another, but such judgment is always mediated by the practitioner's own cultural presuppositions.

Medical anthropologist and physician Paul Farmer documents suffering in a number of locations, including Haiti. Farmer notes that the suffering associated with structural violence can seem almost invisible.

---

25. Scheper-Hughes, *Death without Weeping*, 269–70.

26. Ibid., 355.

One of the reasons for this invisibility is the exoticization of suffering, which allows us to distance ourselves from suffering that is more remote from our own lives. He writes that the sheer weight of suffering makes it difficult to describe, since facts and numbers objectify the victims. The dynamics and distribution of suffering are poorly understood. Individual case studies of people give us insight into suffering, but they must be read against the backdrop of culture, history, and political economy. Farmer believes that liberation theology does a better job of attempting to understand the suffering along with social analysis than many theologies or philosophies. He warns against the tendency to confuse structural violence with cultural difference, which is one form of essentialism used to explain away suffering by suggesting that certain practices are just "part of the culture." Suffering, he argues, is universal, but not all suffering is equal. Uncovering the hidden suffering and attending to it and to the context that surrounds it is a task that he feels should be given priority.[27]

RESPONDING TO SUFFERING AS A PROFESSIONAL

A variety of skills are necessary for the professional regard of suffering. Professionals are expected to regard suffering in the context of an individual's life and with an appreciation for the intercultural differences that might shape that suffering. Professionals also need to maintain a balance between imagining the suffering as if it were their own and regarding it without being destroyed by empathic overload.

Each profession has a history of regarding suffering and expected responses to that suffering. Helga Kuhse describes the history of nineteenth-century nursing as subservience based on two metaphors, namely, nurse as helpmate and nurse as dutiful soldier.[28] The gender division in regarding suffering and finding its cause meant that professions valued different aspects of this professional regard. Doctors focused on the symptom and remained emotionally detached while diagnosing the problem and deciding on the treatment.

William Hurt, in his role as a highly skilled surgeon in the film *The Doctor* (1991), exemplifies technically proficient but joking detachment as he makes fun of colleagues, patients, and medical students in the course of his workday. His manner changes radically when he finds

27. Farmer, *Pathologies of Power*, 40.

28. Kuhse, *Caring*, chapter 2.

himself a patient. He chastises medical students for referring to patients by their diagnoses rather than by their names.

When regarding suffering, how can one manage the emotional challenge while simultaneously offering competent care? Halpern argues that by learning how to empathize, "physicians gain access to a source of understanding illness and suffering that can make them more effective healers."[29] In order to empathize accurately, physicians need to be self-aware and avoid projection of their own unacknowledged emotions onto patients. Nursing literature describes ways of knowing for nurses that include "personal knowing." This type of knowledge depends on reflection and perspective-taking that acknowledges the other as subject rather than object.[30]

WESTERN MEDICINE

Technical superiority and caring can sometimes be interpreted as being in opposition to each other. Western medicine is often presented as more detached, objective, and rational than other forms of medicine. High degrees of specialization allow Western medicine to offer specialized expertise on, for example, the bones of the hand. Such specialized knowledge privileges knowledge over empathy and may or may not be accompanied by caring on the part of the professional.

Alternative forms of care, such as shiatsu, osteopathy, and Reiki place empathy at the forefront of the diagnostic process through a highly skilled form of listening. Although the presenting symptom or source of suffering may be located in the hand, the practitioner considers all the meanings of that source and its interconnection to other parts of the body that may be triggering that suffering or participating in that pain.

The professional culture and context of society affects how one regards suffering; judgments can be so much a part of the professional culture that the individual practitioner may not even be aware of them. Kleinman observes that "the Western tradition's emphasis on the subjective feelings of the afflicted individual, often viewed as isolated and forlorn, is the dominant analytic paradigm for understanding the suffering that results from chronic illness and disability."[31] The range of

29. Halpern, *From Detached Concern*, xi.

30. Jacobs, "Personal Knowing," 23–28.

31. Kleinman, *Writing at the Margin*, 163.

socially acceptable suffering from certain conditions and diseases excludes others, resulting in individuals suffering alone. Those contemplating or undergoing sexual reassignment or transgender surgery, for example, often find themselves extremely isolated, lonely, and lacking social support. Conditions with social stigma lack the resources that are accorded other diseases; when a disease becomes a cause, however, the situation can change.

Suffering challenges our perception and expectation of the good life. We do not care to be reminded that life can change in an instant. Death and all the stages of suffering that might precede it are too difficult to imagine. Even health care professionals who daily confront various manifestations of illness and suffering find it easier to keep that suffering at a distance than to imagine being in the client's place. Imagining that place is, however, a key step in engaging empathy, as we will see further on.

Regarding suffering is not limited to health care professions; it is a challenge for many helping professions. Teachers, for example, are faced daily with the suffering of children and adults whose context has shaped their ability to learn. Young children of immigrant parents arrive at their neighborhood schools, and teachers are expected to deal with their varying levels of readiness for school. As a child, I was brought to the local kindergarten with few English language skills. The teacher, nearing the end of her career, had no patience for the extra work involved in making me "school-ready." I remember spending many hours consigned to a corner where I wept quietly in utter misery. For that teacher, an immigrant child was an exception; in many schools today, particularly in the cities, a diverse classroom has become the norm. However, the needs of some displaced and refugee people are enormous, and those who seek to help them will likely confront overwhelming suffering.

CHANGES IN DISEASE, DETECTION, AND DECISIONS

New diseases and new cures punctuate the history of medicine, and social stigma attached to new or old forms of disease and suffering are socially constructed. William McNeill's study of the history of plagues provides a historical overview of society's reception of different diseases and the suffering they engender.[32] Historians of health or medicine have

32. McNeill, *Plagues and Peoples*.

studied one specific disease, such as the history of cholera or tuberculosis, or broader concepts, such as disease prevention, sanitation, or public health. The outbreak of a new disease or the sudden occurrence of a natural disaster exposes conflicts in social values and priorities. Maureen O'Connell examines the aftermath of Hurricane Katrina and the conflicting values towards the poor that hindered an effective response.[33] New technologies and innovative treatments simultaneously offer hope for the eradication of suffering and create new complexities and ethical dilemmas. Screening increases early detection, but in the case of prenatal care, it forces individuals and society to confront their notions of the kinds of lives they feel are worth preserving.

Disability advocates argue for a more inclusive definition of normal. Thomas Reynolds expands the notion of hospitality to include those most vulnerable.[34] Advances in medical care have increased the life expectancy of those with certain diseases but created new suffering related to their unexpected survivorship. Suffering is thus continually being redefined, with newly framed cultural expectations. Mel Haberman observes that cancer is being redefined as a chronic, life-threatening disease rather than a terminal disease. Although patients are considered cancer-free, a normal response to survivorship is called chronic sorrow.[35] Sheila Santacroce and Ya-Ling Lee have examined post-traumatic stress symptoms (PTSS) in young adult survivors of childhood cancer. Adaptation requires careful communication between survivor and practitioner to address the complex issues that surround survivorship.[36]

LEARNING TO REGARD SUFFERING

The professional regard of suffering is filtered through the practitioner's personal experiences of suffering. Although many students feel the need to disconnect their personal histories from their clinical experiences, such detachment does not result in a completely objective stance towards patients. Some personal experiences may increase a practitioner's ability to understand a client, whereas others might make a client's scenario too close for comfort.

33. O'Connell, *Compassion*.

34. Reynolds, *Vulnerable Communion*.

35. Haberman, "Suffering and Survivorship," 121–42.

36. Santacroce and Lee, "Uncertainty, Posttraumatic Stress," 259–66.

A practitioner who is a breast cancer survivor may have a great deal of empathy for someone who has had the same experiences. If, however, the patient has been diagnosed with further metastases, the encounter may bring many fears to the surface for the practitioner and cause a great deal of discomfort. Practitioners who are themselves parents of young children may find certain clinical situations almost unbearable.

A practitioner may have little patience or empathy for a patient who has contributed to ill health through self-destructive practices. In fact, such discriminatory practices on the part of practitioners can contribute to stigmatization and moral blaming. This is particularly true when a patient is seen as suffering from chronic lifestyle diseases, such as lung cancer resulting from smoking. Professionals may hold judgmental attitudes towards specific populations, such as the homeless, or towards specific illnesses, such as diabetes or hepatitis B, or to patients who are obese, addicted, or labeled noncompliant. Transforming deeply held prejudices and judgments requires educational interventions through transformative learning, which allows the practitioner to see clients in all the complexities of their circumstances and the suffering that encompasses them (see chapter 5). Empathy is a key element in observing the other and in recognizing the experience and suffering of the other without judgment.

ACKNOWLEDGING SUFFERING AND ANSWERING WHY

According to theologian Douglas John Hall, acknowledging the reality of suffering is the first step in being able to enter into the suffering of others.[37] By extension, ignoring individual suffering will close the door on developing a patient-practitioner relationship or constrain it to such an extent that patients cannot authentically share their situation with the observer. Regarding suffering also challenges us to examine how we have responded to our own suffering in personal and professional contexts and how to reconstruct the way our experiences and beliefs have shaped that response. Without this personal work of reviewing one's beliefs, the practitioner may be unaware of the blocks that inhibit full understanding of the other.

Several years ago, I worked as a research nurse on an epidemiological study of congenital defects in infants. The target population of the

---

37. Hall, *God and Human Suffering*, 140–41.

study was children aged six months or less who had been born with a birth defect. My initial contact with the parents explained the study and asked for their participation in an interview. To do the interview, I traveled to their homes, within a geographic range of no more than four hours from the city in which I lived. I visited women in urban high rises and housing projects, suburban homes, farms, and cottages. In most cases, their lives were changed from the moment they gave birth. When I arrived at each home, I was never sure if the child was still alive or if the defect had been so severe that the infant might have died shortly after birth. In the first few moments in each home, I knew that I had to quickly establish trust. Uniformly, the parents were desperate for answers to the questions "Why me?" and "Why this child?" Those were, of course, the questions that I was unable to answer and had been trained to deflect. As a blind interviewer, I had no inside information to the study, so I could not even express an opinion as to why the defect had happened. Some women were concerned about health issues in their community, particularly when they believed there was an environmental cause. Others felt isolated in their experience of having a child with a defect.

I often wished I could give mothers an answer that would allow them to settle the *why* questions—questions that would persist for many of them for years as they struggled to balance this inexplicable reality with their own sense of responsibility.

Illness or suffering disrupts ordinary life and focuses the attention of clients and families on questions such as, "Why me?", "Why now?", or "What for?" When asked these questions by patients, many health care professionals view them as unanswerable and outside of their expertise. Part of being able to hear and respond to such questions requires helping professionals to deal with their own spiritual questions, and also to be comfortable with the diverse range of questions and answers that are held by an increasingly pluralistic world. If professional students have not done such personal work prior to their professional education, it is important that such reflection be encouraged by the curriculum. Such reflection must be unfolded in an atmosphere of trust and acceptance, providing students with safety and confidentiality. This encounter with deep differences is a transformative learning task that requires mentoring and support as new understandings become integrated into one's habit of mind.[38]

38. Curry-Stevens, "New Forms," 48.

PARKER PALMER AND REGARDING SUFFERING

Educator Parker Palmer described his experience with depression and the various types of assistance he received from his well-intentioned friends. When one group of friends attempted to commiserate by saying, "I know exactly how you feel," Palmer tuned out the rest of their conversation. He could no longer hear their words because they were false and made him feel even more isolated. By contrast, one friend provided exactly what he needed when he arrived almost daily to sit in silence with him and to massage his feet.

The challenge in being present a suffering person is to "simply stand respectfully at the edge of that person's mystery and misery. Standing there, we feel useless and powerless, which is exactly how a depressed person feels—and our unconscious need as Job's comforters is to reassure ourselves that we are not like the sad soul before us."[39] The posture of silent attention and waiting is a necessary moment in the extension of empathic regard.

NARRATIVE

In *The Diving Bell and the Butterfly*, successful magazine editor Jean-Dominique Bauby describes locked-in syndrome, which he experienced after a stroke left his body paralyzed but his mind completely aware. His memoir was dictated to an assistant using an abbreviated code based on the blink of his eyelid, the only body part over which he had any control. Such a memoir disrupts our sense of how life should go. Bauby had enjoyed a privileged and comfortable life; with little warning, his life was turned upside down. All his relationships were affected—relationships with his body, his family, and his future.[40] Illness narratives such as these can help to engage practitioners and students with suffering in ways that facilitate reflection and empathy.

Listening to such a story in person can establish the beginning of an empathic professional relationship. Rita Charon notes that when patients tell stories of their illnesses, they are "revealing aspects of self closest to the skin thus obliging practitioners morally to listen to the lives of others."[41] Memoir can provide one way to open the discussion

39. Palmer, *Let Your Life Speak*, 62–63.
40. Bauby, *Diving Bell and the Butterfly*.
41. Charon, *Narrative Medicine*, 78.

of illness experience to practitioners and to engage their imagination with questions like, "What would someone like Bauby experience?" or "How would I cope with such a loss of independence?" By reading a patient narrative using the imagination, one "relinquishes one's own coherent experience of the world for another's unexpected, unexplored, unplumbed, potentially volatile viewpoint."[42]

Fiction can also provide insight into human responses to suffering. In recent years, popular fiction books such as *The Shack* have struck a chord with readers who struggle to find meaning in suffering. In *The Shack*, a father attempts to come to terms with the kidnapping and death of his child by engaging in conversation with a God who challenges his preconceived notions of both God and the nature of forgiveness.[43]

Elie Wiesel's exploration of evil in his book *Night* continues to challenge readers to understand how such things could happen and to ensure that they are not forgotten.[44] Fiction does not require that the reader has had the same experience of losing a child or experiencing genocide to be able to imagine the nature of the suffering described. Reading or listening allows one to experience alternate visions of reality and trains the imagination to expand from what it knows concretely to what it can imagine. This ability is essential to empathy, since empathy relies on the imagination to provide insight into the other.

Reluctance to regard the suffering of individuals or communities creates an inauthentic situation for professionals. This is because ignoring the suffering in favor of treatment leads to disconnection in the aims of treatment and in the potential relationality of the situation. As Charon observes, the ability to hear the suffering of another means that one has confronted and found at least provisional answers to life's big questions. Some students might have addressed such questions before entering professional school as a result of personal illness or family circumstance. Others discover, during their education, the prevalence of suffering and the limits of available treatments to relieve that suffering. Education should offer the opportunity for students to be mentored and accompanied through their experiences of witnessing suffering regardless of their previous personal experience with suffering.

42. Ibid., 112.
43. Young, *The Shack*.
44. Wiesel, *Night*.

Can the conversation about suffering at any level explore both what unites human experience and what is experienced differently? How have various cultural, religious and spiritual traditions attempted to respond to the issue of suffering, and how has art, ritual, and liturgy embodied a response to that suffering? How can professionals learn to respond to the big questions of suffering, while dealing with individual and family instances of that suffering? Meaningful engagement with practices of different traditions related to care of the sick person, care of the body, and care of the dying person allows the helping professional to encounter the diversity of beliefs in a pluralistic world. In addition to cultural differences, students in helping professions will also meet those for whom their traditions no longer speak meaningfully and who are essentially homeless in a spiritual sense. As part of the professional training, one must engage with the spiritual questions personally in order to be able to hear and meet the needs of suffering clients. Meaningful questions that will challenge the helping professional might include the following:

1. Why me?

2. Why now?

3. What can be done?

4. Will things ever be the same?

5. Will others still care about me if I am changed in various ways?

6. What hope can I have in this situation?

7. Where will I find the courage or resources to deal with this?

8. What will the rest of my life be like?

9. What will happen to me if this treatment or intervention does not work?

10. What happens to me when I die?

11. Who will care?

Perhaps one way to sort out the *why* questions is into two categories: (1) questions about the human condition and (2) questions related to where to find hope in the face of that knowledge. The first category of *why* questions can be answered from a variety of philosophical, theological, comparative religious, or psychological perspectives. The notion of hope, however, is complex, since most helping professionals are careful to balance presenting false hope with clinical realities. In the past, professionals believed it was acceptable to lie to the patient in order to preserve hope. Hope for clients with chronic conditions requires a re-framing of one's expectations and requires transformation at the deepest levels. Hope and trust are spiritual concepts that can affect health promotion and health-affirming choices in clients. Sally Thorne has studied the role of communication between patients and health-care providers and has argued that communication can facilitate "coping, self-care management, and an optimal quality of life for those with chronic illness."[45]

The stress on positive thinking in combating certain illnesses shifts blame to patients who do not show the heroic courage that many survivors exhibit. A practitioner may personally believe that a patient's prognosis is grave or hopeless, but may later be surprised by an unexpected remission or healing.

The professional regard towards suffering may include an admission that mystery and uncertainty can allow for unexplained interruptions of the course of illness. That uncertainty may be ascribed to the randomness of the universe or to the intervention of divine forces of healing, but openness to different perspectives that allows for empathic regard. For some, these interventions can be encouraged by the use of prayer, laying on of hands, meditation, complementary or alternative medicine, massage, music, art therapy, or therapeutic touch.[46] A practitioner's ability to be open to a patient's choice of these types of alternatives may affect how much the patient is willing to share about his or her beliefs and experiences.

REFLECTING ON POSSIBLE ANSWERS

Suffering triggers questions that draw us into the diversity of other beliefs and answers. Most world religions address the notion of suffering and the meaning of life. Individual responses to such answers vary widely Philosophers, novelists, artists, and musicians respond to suffering in ways that speak the unspeakable and can provide solace to those who feel alone in their experience. For practitioners who will regard suffering throughout their careers, a broad exposure to both explanations of suffering and creative responses to it through the arts will be essential parts

45. Thorne, "Shifting Images of Chronic Illness," 173–78.
46. See Sperry, *Spirituality in Clinical Practice*, chapter 7.

of their professional training. Some faculties have created space in the formal curriculum for social, cultural, and religious aspects of suffering and encourage exposing students to the arts as a way to generate reflection and perspective on their experiences.

Robert Smith describes three aspects of the religious response to suffering (of either individuals or communities) that exist across cultures. These include the intellectual dimension, ethical dimension, and experiential dimension. The intellectual dimension includes a search for meaning. The ethical dimension "often occurs as a set of questions about how to respond to the threat of personal disintegration."[47] Helping people sort through their own understanding of the moral understanding of suffering requires great respect for both diversity of belief and flexibility for change in a person's understanding over time. The experiential aspect of suffering is the experience that the person must pass through, which will lead to a different understanding of self and of life. Although suffering in this dimension can be ultimately transformative, everyone does not necessarily experience it in that way.

WORLD RELIGIONS

Most of the major world religions address the nature and purpose of suffering. John Bowker analyzes how suffering is explained in Judaism, Christianity, Islam, Marxism, Hinduism, and Buddhism.[48] However, understanding a belief system does not illumine how individuals live out those beliefs in their daily experience, particularly when disrupted by the experience of suffering. Sacred texts or scriptures can provide the basis for ongoing interpretation. Authorities who are acquainted with the history of the texts and their reading provide learned commentary on the texts. Suffering sometimes brings a closer encounter with those texts, with enhanced understanding of the meaning of suffering.

Each religion recommends practices for the faithful, which may include showing compassion or care for the neighbor or stranger, practicing forgiveness, or working for justice. A moral stance can be deduced from different religions that inform how one is to live life while on earth. Most religions are further distinguished by different schools of thought or denominations that have specific histories, traditions, and interpreta-

47. Smith, "Theological Perspectives," 159–72.

48. Bowker, *Problems of Suffering.*

tions of beliefs. In full acknowledgment of the complexity of those belief systems, it is beyond the scope of this book to do more than introduce the student to the notion of religions and spirituality in order to better understand some of the answers to the question, "What is suffering, and where does it originate?"

The question of suffering was placed at the heart of Buddhism when its founder Gautama (c.566–c.480 BC) asked, "Why do pain and suffering exist?" The Buddha teaches that suffering in its "universal and existential state can be fought, first and foremost, by recognizing it."[49]

Suffering has been translated as *dukkha*, meaning intolerable or unsustainable. The nature of suffering in Buddhism has two principle aspects. The first is the practical side, namely, the inevitable experience of every man, woman, and child; the second aspect of suffering is philosophical—why does one suffer?[50] There is no permanent self in Buddhism, since the individual is composed of changing physical or mental forces that can be divided into five aggregates. The five aggregates include the four great elements (our five senses), sensations derived from contact with the world, perceptions, mental formations, and consciousness. These five groups constitute the "I" and are constantly changing.

The Four Noble Truths are central to Buddhism and include the following: all is suffering, suffering is caused by desire or attachment, eliminating desire/attachment will eliminate suffering, and the Noble Eight-fold path can eliminate desire/attachment. The Eight-fold path includes holding to right views, right intent, right speech, right conduct, right livelihood, right effort, right mindfulness, and right concentration.

The Theravada tradition of Buddhism teaches that everyone must individually seek salvation through his or her own efforts. To attain nirvana, one must relinquish earthly desires and live a monastic life. The Mahayana tradition teaches that salvation comes through the grace of bodhisattvas. Bodhisattvas defer their own enlightenment to help others, thus enabling many more living beings to attain salvation. The seeker hopes to reach nirvana, which is a state in which there are no desires and no individual consciousness, but one in which suffering ends. The end of suffering or *dukkha* is also then the end of craving. Suffering is not to be avoided but is part of the path to nirvana. Realizing the truths of death and chance allows the individual to attain enlightenment.

49. Lampert, *Traditions of Compassion*, xviii.
50. Selles, "Concept of Dukkha."

According to Islamic belief, suffering can be attributed to the power of sin or the testing by God of an individual. Sin can be forgiven, and reconciliation is possible. Islam teaches one to endure suffering with hope and faith. We are not counseled to resist it, or to ask why. Instead, we accept it as God's will and live through it with faith that God never asks more of us than we can endure. However, Islam also teaches us to work actively to alleviate the suffering of others. Recognizing that we are the cause of our own suffering, we work to bring suffering to an end. In the Islamic view, righteous individuals are revealed through patient acceptance of their own suffering and through their good works for others. And if we are suffering as a consequence of our own unbelief, then good works will relieve our pain.[51]

Suffering is an essential component of life in the Hindu belief system, wherein each person is accountable for his or her actions. That is the basis of Karma. Our lives at any given point are a net result of our past actions, both good and evil. We are capable of good as well as evil, since God gave us intelligence and independence. Therefore, we are responsible for the consequences of our actions. The Hindu belief system also includes the belief that our soul, which is immortal, goes through endless life cycles and somehow carries with it an imprint of our past actions. Therefore, the suffering of a good person can be the result of actions in past lives. When a person suffers in this life, they are paying their debt back to the universe to bring balance back to the circle of life. One can experience less suffering in the next life by doing acts of good in the present. Hindus believe their position in life is based on their actions in a previous life, or lives: This is the Law of Karma, which states that from good must come good, and from evil must come evil. Hinduism embraces the existence of suffering in the world and in doing so teaches the paths for one to be free of suffering and obtain *moksha*, which means freedom or liberation, which is the ultimate human goal.

In one of the schools of Hindu thought, the *Samkhya* system, pain can be described as threefold: originating from the sufferer, from created beings, and from the gods. Pain is located within the very nature of things. The potential pain or pain yet to come is called the purpose of life. Suffering in the form of pain, decay, and death are common to human experience but do not form the sum total of reality.

51. For discussions of suffering in Islam, see Koslowski, *Origins and Overcoming of Evil*. See also Heemskerk, *Suffering in Mutazilite Theology*.

The permanent cessation of pain cannot be brought about by thought, but rather by *moksha*. The individual experiences three kinds of suffering: from internal causes, from physical or material causes, and from circumstances. The way out of suffering is through right knowledge that destroys ignorance and replaces it with understanding. Through the process of liberation, the false self is shed and the true self comes into being. Suffering is not then part of the soul but part of the false self or ego. First, *dukkha* is revealed to have a redemptive quality; it functions as a guide to knowledge that will end suffering. Second, *dukkha* is connected to a state of ignorance that leads one to place ultimate importance in the physical body or the immediate. Third, one can eventually escape suffering.[52] Unlike the explanation of a "fall" into sin, *Samkhya* argues that all is as it always was. Suffering is part of the objective reality of the world and has always been so (*prakriti*). The universe also contains *purusa* that is unchanging and neutral, both free from pain and pleasure. Discrimination allows one to distinguish *prakriti* from *purusa*. The path to knowledge is attained through detachment and meditation.

Although specific doctrines might change, several themes are common to many world religions. Religion describes the role of the self and the other and how they are related to each other. Such religious beliefs can also teach one how to live in the present reality with compassion for the self and the other. Lessons are provided in how to regard human failure and willingness to change. The role of illusion in Buddhism is important, warning the individual to regard present reality as passing. Finally, the centrality of compassion underscores the importance of kindness to the stranger.

Many patients carry unexamined or inherited beliefs about suffering that are attributed to Christian beliefs but that represent misunderstandings of the nature of suffering and the hope of the gospel. Patients may believe that God is punishing them through the illness experience or that they should somehow choose suffering as part of their education. Choosing suffering or inflicting suffering as some pedagogical exercise is not an acceptable interpretation of Christian doctrine. Religion does not exempt us from the realities of human life—suffering and death are parts of that life. Belief in a future where suffering and death will no longer dominate our lives is part of the promises of Christian faith. The literature on the meaning of suffering is vast and well covered elsewhere.

52. Selles, "Concept of Dukkha."

Professional students need to be introduced to the literature on suffering from both a religious studies and a social scientific perspective. Such reading will enable them to put into perspective their own experiences of suffering, but also to develop empathic regard for others who suffer or who understand their suffering differently. An understanding of pastoral practices in relation to care of the body in illness, health, and death, as well as ritual and liturgical practice, can only improve professional practice and the ability to empathize.

In addition to the answers given by theologians, philosophers, and other thinkers, the patient perspective allows us to see how some of these ideas are lived out in the lives of patients and clients. In a study of the responses of children and their families to children's cancer symptoms, R. L. Woodgate and L. F. Degner examine how patients regard suffering when it is seen as part of the necessary regimen towards finding a cure.[53]

Patients and clients with established belief systems and those who have never closely examined their beliefs find ways to deal with their hopes and fears in practical ways that may include contradictions between belief and practice, faith and confidence in an unseen future, or denial of previously held beliefs. Such transitions and adaptations to the power of suffering in individuals and communities are important to the course of their illness and to their participation in activities that support or detract from wholeness.

SUFFERING AS COMMUNAL CHALLENGE

Suffering has been the target of many platitudes that are largely unhelpful to those experiencing suffering. Yet suffering presents the greatest challenge to human individuals and communities, namely the challenge to be present to those suffering. As part of the human reality on earth, we have an active role to play in regarding suffering. Douglas John Hall notes, "In whatever ways God continues to suffer with those who suffer—and they are numberless—we for our part know that this is our vocation. We are part of the response of God to the massive suffering of God's

---

53. Woodgate and Degner, "Expectations and Beliefs about Children's Cancer," 479–91.

world."[54] Such an active role requires a willingness to experience pain and to stand with those who are alone in challenging situations.

For those who share diverse religious beliefs, that challenge means forming not communities of comfort and like-mindedness, but communities of suffering. Hall notes that gathering as a suffering community and sharing burdens is the beginning of the healing process. He contrasts this active participation in suffering to a passive "spectator spirituality" that exists in a suffering world "without passion or compassion." Although the concept of rejoicing in suffering has often been both unattainable and misrepresented, Hall says that the source of rejoicing in suffering is not due to evidence of personal redemption but because it points "towards a hope for *our world*."[55]

Liberation theologian Jon Sobrino defines mercy as the basic attitude toward the suffering of another whereby one reacts to eradicate that suffering for the sole reason that it exists. We do not have the option to turn away in the face of suffering because the suffering of another challenges our being. Action responds to the belief that the suffering of another ought not to be. Mercy, in Sobrino's definition, is not just the work of the individual, but also of the church, whose job it is to be with the suffering other. He describes the recognition of suffering and the response of compassion as something pre-theological and even pre-religious. The elimination of suffering from the world is the priority.[56]

On the subject of suffering, Dorothee Soelle notes that suffering people must find a way to express their experiences rather than having someone speak on their behalf. She challenges us to work to abolish the circumstances that lead to suffering, including poverty and political tyranny. Suffering, she notes, affects every dimension of life. Her critique of traditional Christian views of suffering targets the notion that, on the one hand, they emphasize divine power, and on the other hand, they highlight the Christian willingness to suffer. The ultimate result of such an understanding merely contributes to Christian masochism, since "suffering is there to break our pride, demonstrate our powerlessness, exploit our dependency. Affliction has the intention of bringing us back to

54. Hall, *God and Human Suffering*, 141.

55. Ibid., 142.

56. Sobrino, *Principle of Mercy*.

a God who only becomes great when he makes us small." [57] She critiques the notion that all suffering is punishment for sin.

Applied to modern faith communities, Soelle's ideas would suggest that the health of a faith community might be measured, not by the budget or the luxury cars in the parking lot, but by its ability to create honest space for members to share their suffering and to stand with the suffering of those outside the walls of the faith community. Rather than hide the pain of brokenness behind smiling faces, members could weep together at the evidence of broken relations around them. Pain therefore leads a person to look outward in order to achieve solidarity. Soelle writes, "The sufferer himself must find a way to express and identify his suffering; it is not sufficient to have someone speak on his behalf. If people cannot speak about affliction they will be destroyed by it, or swallowed up by apathy."[58]

These approaches to suffering challenge us find connections between sufferers and observers and to enter willingly into a place of deep attentiveness and listening. Choosing to enter into suffering is a far more challenging task than blaming the victims or isolating them from the others. This task of *mit-leiden*, or suffering with, is not restricted to professionals, or to faith communities, but is part of our human responsibility to recognize the interconnectedness of our life on earth. If professional students do not encounter what Giroux has called a "pedagogy of responsibility," how can they be expected to work out of a politics of commitment?[59]

SUFFERING IN ACUTE OR CHRONIC SITUATIONS

Cassell distinguishes disease from illness, with diseases being specific entities characterized by disturbances in the structure or function of any part, organ, or system of the body. By contrast, illnesses affect the whole person and are the set of "disordered functions, body sensations, and feelings by which persons know themselves to be unwell." [60] Although a chronic disease may be present, one cannot assume that the person is suffering from chronic illness. In some cases, disease may be absent but

---

57. Soelle, *Suffering*, 19.

58. Ibid., 76.

59. Giroux, "Cultural Studies, Public Pedagogy," 59–79.

60. Cassell, *Nature of Suffering*, 49.

the pain may still be disabling, as in chronic pain syndrome, for example. In a sense, his work highlights the individual nature of suffering. It is an important reminder for professionals that despite our knowledge about the expected course of illness or the normal and abnormal limits that are expected, we must leave room for individual variations and experiences. Professionals who lack the necessary humility forget that patients' experiences are their own, and expertise in a professional field does not automatically provide one with precise insight into patients' experiences. For this, one must practice empathic regard, attempting to view the patient's experience from within, rather than impose generalized understandings on that experience.

ANTHROPOLOGY OF SUFFERING

Global suffering has many names, including torture and genocide as intentional forms of harm. In addition, "unintended" harm is done by globalization, unequal distribution of resources, exploitation, and disregard for ecological questions. Only by understanding local suffering and its relation to global inequities can one accurately confront the suffering of the world's poor or marginalized.

Although it is a challenge for an outsider to describe the experience of suffering in other cultures, there are common elements that transcend culture. Professionals who work with suffering populations or individuals could benefit from anthropological understandings of how people suffer and the diverse cultural meanings of that suffering. To respond effectively to the diverse populations who seek help, such intercultural understanding will be an essential skill. The ability to contextualize suffering is an essential prerequisite to effective and empathic response.

CONCLUSION: REGARDING SUFFERING

Witnessing suffering is a difficult task for many. Observers report being exhausted, drained, or emotionally challenged when placed face-to-face with a suffering person. The desire to fix the situation, alleviate the pain, or change the conditions that led to the pain can overwhelm the observer. Identification with the sufferer can lead the observer to experience similar pain. For some observers, awkwardness and the inability to find an appropriate response can trigger emotional or physical withdrawal. In addition, practitioners are simultaneously learning to complete a procedure, deal with technology, reassure family, appear more skilled than they are, and deal with their own anxieties in these situations.

For beginning practitioners, it may be easier to focus on the technology, or on the specific injury, wound, or procedure, than it is to relate to the patient's suffering in the situation. Although the student may be learning to start an IV, the patient has not only that moment to deal with, but also the cumulated effects of all the previous procedures, pain, and uncertainty that accompany that experience. Because the suffering is subjective and individual, a professional might choose to focus on the technique or procedure rather than the suffering. The patient's side of this encounter likely includes the memory of past suffering, whereas time for the clinician is often experienced as discrete events that need to be done under intense pressure. Notions of time and suffering are shaped by the professional culture and the client experience of suffering, and they may be marked in very different ways.

Student practitioners in health settings may panic when they witness for the first time a post-surgical complication, an acute myocardial infarction, a woman in childbirth, or a patient in deep depression. A profound sense of inadequacy and incompetence can accompany such experiences. Often the student attempts to compensate for such identification by assuming a detached professional role. Mentors can either provide space and time for the examination of these complex emotions or choose to shut down discussion completely.[61] Such a choice will have important consequences for the professional student in the future.

Regarding suffering is not enough. Margaret Farley notes that compassion is a powerful response to human need and suffering. Sometimes, however, an appeal to compassion can remain an empty appeal—not because the experience of compassion is empty but because the recognition of what compassion requires is missing. Further, Farley reminds us that compassion needs to be normatively shaped.[62] Farley calls for an attitude of compassionate respect that recognizes that care has normative requirements. Care has several meanings, including a disposition to affective response, affective response itself, and actions that express affective response. The determinants of right caring, she notes, depend on the reality of the cared for as well as the carer, and the nature of the relationship governs what kind of caring happens.

61. Angoff, "Crying in the Curriculum," 1017–18.
62. Farley, Compassionate Respect, 64.

Learning how to be present with the suffering client requires learning and experience. Kleinman observes, "Perhaps this is an aspect of physicianhood that is so deeply indwelling that it cannot be taught didactically, that it must be learned through the difficult experiences of the student's own pain and the pressing need to do good for others. Perhaps it is also dependent on the practitioner's current stage of adult development. Can one effectively empathize and assist another person's grief, if one has not personally experienced bereavement? Perhaps nothing short of the personal reality of illness or doctoring can fashion this wisdom."[63]

Although we cannot and would not seek to experience all that our clients or students experience—indeed, it would be far too great a burden to do so—empathy allows the practitioner to gain insight by standing in the "as if" position with the suffering person. Taking a moment to experience this reality and to stand with the suffering other is preliminary to responding to that suffering, either with the respect that Farley describes, or through the act of bearing witness. In the next chapter, we will examine the process of bearing witness as a professional's response to the suffering of others.

---

63. Kleinman, *Ilness Narrative*, 251.

QUESTIONS FOR FURTHER DISCUSSION

1. Describe an experience where you witnessed suffering. Describe the feelings you had at the time. Recall what you said or did at the time.

2. Describe an experience of your own suffering. What were the things that made the experience better or worse for you? Do you prefer isolation, or do you seek out others?

3. The media is filled with stories of social suffering. Research one such location of suffering. What factors contribute to this suffering? What sources of assistance have been provided? When you read the media coverage, do you feel empathy for these people, or do you feel detached? Describe your feelings.

4. When you have experienced suffering in your family or among friends, what was their response to you? Describe an experience of suffering from your childhood.

5. As a child, what explanations were you given for suffering? What explanations do you currently give to explain suffering?

6. Do you belong to any organizations or faith communities that respond to the suffering in the world? What types of response do they provide?

7. Have you ever experienced healing space? What, for you, are the characteristics of healing space? Can you draw or describe it?

8. Have you participated in rituals or liturgies that respond to suffering? Describe the ritual and how it made you feel.

9. Choose one art form (film, novel, poetry, music) that deals with suffering. Write a short reflection on how the piece engaged with suffering and how it affected you.

10. Visit a faith community and observe how its practices engage with suffering. Journal or blog a short reflection on your observations as an outsider or guest in this community.

4

Bearing Witness

What we can learn already from oral history and trauma studies is that the work of bearing witness does not do violence to the speaker, does not *interfere* in the telling, but rather is committed to active, respectful, confirming listening.[1]

INTRODUCTION

I WORKED AS A per-diem nurse in a suburban group home for adults with physical and intellectual disabilities. One of my regular clients was Marie.[2] Her few possessions included some street clothes and institutional pajamas. She was autistic and had spent decades in an institution. She did not communicate in any discernible way and preferred to stay in her room. I tried to connect with her through singing, speaking, and talking in her native language, but I never observed a response.

My other client was Stan, a man in his sixties who was surprisingly robust considering that he had been bedridden for years. Caring for him included placing him on a lift and taking him to the whirlpool bath. He also received feeding by stomach tube, medications, and passive exercises to his limbs. Stan would make some sounds, perhaps in protest, in response to treatment, but he did not communicate in a way that might be called interactive or intentional.

The care of Stan, Marie, and others in a state-funded group home was compassionate and followed state regulations. Staff continued to communicate with the clients even if the communication appeared to be one-sided. These clients had spent a large proportion of their lives in state institutions and had been moved out to smaller, homelike settings

---

1. Charon, *Narrative Medicine*, 180–81.
2. Client names have been changed.

as a result of de-institutionalization policies. The staff of the group home acted as both family and friends to these clients, who had no other caregivers or family and who could not survive without this care.

The staff did its best to create a safe and secure home environment for these vulnerable clients. In doing so, the professional caregivers were first of all witnesses to the vulnerability and sometimes the suffering of these residents. In order to be an effective advocate and practitioner, it is first of all necessary to provide technically competent care, and second, to be a witness to suffering, recognizing and respecting the vulnerability "as if" it were one's own. The clients in this group home had been de-institutionalized after decades in state hospitals. Their own narratives had been interrupted, broken, and lost. The charts at the group home kept careful record of their daily care but had no history. Although Marie was from Quebec, there was no record of how she had ended up in suburban Connecticut. No family or friends came to visit Marie and Stan. The staff at the group home was their only family. Whether they thought about the past or worried about the future was impossible to know. Life for them was a series of present moments.

The key to understanding witness is that the relationship is dialogical and dyadic even when the client cannot express his or her experience. Yet in situations where one bears either active or passive witness, one must always be aware of the privilege that separates one's own voice from the voiceless. Professionals have power, education, resources, networks, and capacities that many of their clients cannot even imagine. The work of justice requires not only a passion for defending the vulnerable and building capacity in those with little, but also a humble reckoning of the immense responsibility of speaking or acting on behalf of others. In this chapter we will examine the notion of bearing witness and look at examples of influential people who used their empathic powers to respond to a perceived need on behalf of others.

In their call to bear witness, individuals become convicted of an injustice. Goodman has studied how people of privilege are often blind to suffering and to their own privilege. Empathy can be a factor in learning to recognize inequities by allowing one to identify with the feelings and the situation of the other. In extending empathic regard, cognitive and affective elements are engaged and may lead to action. Dehumanization can reduce empathy and allow one to regard the other as less human and even deserving of lesser treatment. Goodman distinguishes between empathy that motivates helping behavior in an individual instance from empathy that supports social activism, working over time to improve conditions.[3]

BEARING WITNESS

The Hebrew Bible describes bearing witness as an act of bringing expert knowledge to a situation. The book of Isaiah describes a judicial process in which deities of other lands are challenged by God to demonstrate their divine status. The passage challenges them to bring their witnesses but continues, "You are my witnesses, says the Lord and my servant whom I have chosen (Isa 43:9–10)."[4] In the New Testament the word "witness" can refer to the act of bearing witness (verb), the activity of witnessing, and the witness that is borne.

The legal sense of bearing witness shifts to include a religious sense of witness. The apostles who were eyewitnesses to the presence of Jesus were confessional witnesses to his life (John 20:28). Another type of witness includes the post-ascension witnesses, such as that of Paul (Acts 22:14–15). In the New Testament, witnessing is first of all concerned with being—you must *be* a witness before you can witness, and the transformation that happens means you cannot help but be empowered to witness.[5]

Such witnessing can depend on affective and cognitive awareness. Henri Nouwen gave up his academic career to live and work at the L'Arche community in Toronto. Nouwen describes a process of being taught by one of the differently-abled clients named Adam, who enabled him to see life in different ways. He writes, "With Adam I knew a sacred presence and I 'saw' the face of God." [6] Adam reminded him that individual accomplishments and competition were not important—what mattered was doing things together. This insight, noted Nouwen, made Adam "the most radical witness to the truth of our lives that I have ever encountered."[7]

3. Goodman, *Promoting Diversity*, 128.

4. *New Oxford Annotated Bible*.

5. Reisinger, "The New Testament Meaning of 'Witness.'"

6. Nouwen, *Adam: God's Beloved*, 53.

7. Ibid., 56.

Being part of this radical witness had its own transformative effects on Nouwen, who left for a period of time to confront his "own abyss." Bearing witness may involve a transformation of those who are the subject of the story and those who would tell it for them. In this case, Adam taught Henri Nouwen, who later wrote the book in which he could bear witness to the truth of the interaction. The encounter was profoundly transformative for Nouwen. In doing daily care for Adam and spending hours in his presence, Nouwen encountered affective, cognitive, and psychomotor domains that caused him to shift previously held beliefs. Adam bore witness that resulted in Nouwen's transformation into one who could later bear witness on Adam's behalf. The ability to bear witness required a conversion that was far greater than an intellectual change in thinking—for Nouwen, this shift occurred on every level of his being.[8]

In a legal context, one can either tell the truth or bear false witness. In a general context, telling a story about an event or a person involves the eyewitness interpreting the event and telling it according to standards of narrative coherence and narrative fidelity.[9] In the telling, events are selected and choices are made to highlight or de-emphasize parts of the narrative. Can the telling ever be completely accurate? Those who would bear witness for others often acknowledge their limitations and their particular perspective, and within those limits they reassert their need to tell the story. When bearing witness is done by a person of privilege on behalf of those who have little, there is always the danger of appropriation.

In his autobiography, Howard Thurman noted that telling a story is always subject to mystery, and no one can enter into the heart of that mystery. Thurman writes, "And this is the strangest of all the paradoxes of the human adventure: we live *inside* all experience, but we are permitted to bear witness only to the *outside*. Such is the riddle of our life and the story of the passing of our days."[10]

Illness stories describe the experience from the inside and allow sick people to reclaim a voice that otherwise is appropriated by the medical establishment. Kleinman gives the term "empathic witnessing"

8. Sperry, *Spirituality in Clinical Practice*, 45. Sperry describes how conversion may include living out changes in all areas of life, including the affective, moral, intellectual, religious, and sociopolitical, as well as the somatic.

9. Fisher, "Narration, Reason, and Community," 307–27.

10. Thurman, *Jesus and the Disinherited*, 270.

to the relational responsibility to be with an ill person "That is the existential commitment to be with the sick person and to facilitate his or her building of an illness narrative."[11] Unlike training in communications techniques, the process of empathic witnessing is not a technique that can be taught, however; it is a moral act that requires relational collaboration between the helping professional and the client.

Illness narratives are a form of resistance to the loss of agency experienced by sick people. Sociologist Arthur Frank contends that patients can resist the reductionist impulses of modern science by bearing witness to their experiences of illness through stories. Stories are not only a way of sharing and creating relationship between the ill person and the observer, but are also a way out of the narrative wreckage that illness can create of one's life. A story that is told truthfully incorporates the chaos that illness creates and becomes witness—reaching beyond the individual to the community.[12] Because story depends on a teller and a listener, it is inherently relational. The dislocation and isolation experienced by a sick person can be overcome through the process of telling and listening.

Scholars have turned to narrative as a way to capture experience—from Holocaust studies in the 1980s through the rise of trauma studies. Both disciplines attempt to honor and bear witness to the experience of survivors. Narrative is a retelling of something that happened (a story). The story has a sequence of events, but the telling or narrative recounts, reorders, and re-emphasizes those events. Narrative can be visual, graphic, or written. Although all cultures engage in story, not all stories are part of our conscious awareness. Stories are transmitted not only through art and literature, but also through inherited memory.

NARRATIVE AND MORAL OBLIGATIONS

Frank describes the interhuman nature of storytelling as narrative ethics that demands both listening and telling. Rita Charon suggests that clients reveal their innermost thoughts related to vulnerability and mortality, and it is the responsibility of practitioners to take time to listen. The privilege of listening extends to teachers, clergy, and others with whom the bond of trust allows for deep sharing. Because illness raises ques-

11. Kleinman, *Ilness Narrative*, 55.

12. Frank, *Wounded Storyteller*, 55–63.

tions of fragility and mortality, when "patients talk about themselves to their doctors or nurses, they are revealing aspects of the self closest to the skin, having pared away the optional layers."[13] Listening demands an act of attention that includes an emptying of self in order to become an instrument for receiving the meaning of another. Active listening in order to be fully present is a learned skill that requires listeners to set aside their concerns in order to receive the reality of the other without judgment.

This emptying is more than mere detachment or removal of the personal from the picture; rather, it is a disciplined, reflective regard. The quality of attention that the practitioner gives the patient honors the story. The emptying of self allows him or her to become an instrument for receiving the meaning of the other. Such emptying may be difficult to imagine in the intense and technology-mediated environments that shape healthcare and education today. The tension and pressure of multiple conflicting commitments are reflected in body language and in a sense of impatience. Interrupting or devaluing the client's story affects both the client and the practitioner, as each are deprived of an opportunity for relational connection.

In her work on educating people from privileged groups, Diane Goodman describes a process of decentering the self that allows one to hear those with less privilege.[14] A listening self that is open to narrative chooses interrelationship over autonomy. The work of bearing witness requires a practitioner who has stood in the face of suffering, recognized personal vulnerability, and made space to listen to the other. Bringing this whole person into the interaction with the other requires a level of personal and professional formation that represents a lifelong challenge, particularly in a professional culture that affirms privilege and power over vulnerable populations. Empathy is an essential ingredient in this challenge to create relationship in the midst of institutions, professional cultures, and reimbursement structures that inhibit the work of caring.

TELLING THE STORY THROUGH THE BODY

The story of suffering is told through the suffering body; in fact, the body bears witness to the story. To split the body from the experience of suf-

---

13. Charon, *Narrative Medicine*, 78.
14. Goodman, *Promoting Diversity and Social Justice*, chapter 3.

fering creates an unnecessary separation that detracts from the overall meaning. Charon underlines the importance of the body in understanding the self when she notes, "At the same time that individuals are able to transcend their definitions by their bodies—such, after all, is the basis for racism, sexism and discrimination against the other-abled—they are also able to incorporate their experience of being embodied into their concept of self and their movement through the world and through life."[15] And the body can refuse to cooperate with the optimistic scripts that are written for it by culture and professional intervention. Theologian Serene Jones notes that optimism about healing in the case of trauma survivors discounts the reality that many reach the end of their life still caught in its "terrifying grip." Jones notes that the body offers a visceral testimony of what has been experienced, but healing can come "in the midst of things." For the professional, presence can offer a steadying support to someone healing from trauma so that together they can move to a new place that allows for an embodied grace.[16]

In the same way that we read fiction to open up new worlds that we have never experienced, listening to a patient's or client's story requires active listening and imagination. The practitioner need not have experienced all that the patient has known and felt—one can listen and imagine the experience "as if" it were one's own. Imaginative listening requires an empathic engagement with the reality of another. Readiness for this type of encounter begins long before one is face to face with a patient—a skill that can be encouraged during professional training. Individual stories emerge with unlimited variation, yet the themes of finding meaning in suffering, yearning for home, and hoping for joy provide melodies that are hauntingly familiar.

PROFESSIONAL PRESENCE

Although listening requires close attention, there are also limits and boundaries to the professional relationship. Perri Klass notes that people who work closely with suffering "must find a way to respond with compassion, imagination, and empathy, but they must respond as professionals, not as friends or family."[17] Recognizing those limits is a skill associated

---

15. Charon, *Narrative Medicine*, 112.

16. Jones, *Trauma and Grace*, 155.

17. Klass, "Empathic Practitioner," 157–70.

with a mature emotional intelligence. As Salovey, Brackett, and Mayer have indicated, it is not enough to have intrapersonal skills, but one must develop interpersonal skills as well. One must recognize the situation of the other, identify the emotions that the client feels, experience emotions in response, and then act or respond appropriately.[18]

Several professions use the term "presence" to describe their task in the face of suffering, and presence can be adapted to fit different professional contexts, including pastoral presence, nursing presence, instrumental friendship, and intersubjective co-presence. Nursing literature refers to transcendence as a possible outcome of the nurse-patient relationship. As a patient deals with a crisis of personal vulnerability, the professional response can be either detachment or transcendence. In this case, transcendence is defined as "the ability to get beyond and outside oneself to perceive, respond to, and be with the sufferer."[19]

Nursing presence has been described as both a quality and a nursing intervention with the potential to facilitate the healing process. Patricia Benner identifies nursing presence under the umbrella of "The Helping Role" as one of the seven domains of nursing practice.[20] Proficiency in application is acquired in the journey from novice to expert clinician. Presence has been described as existential in scope. This most demanding aspect of caring requires a lifetime of practice and is communicated through a touch, a tone, a glance, or a state of silent immersion as the nurse seeks to understand the patient's situation by coexisting and co-creating in the moment. Not only does this skill help to establish trust in the nurse-patient dyad, but it also contributes to the nurse's mental well-being, satisfaction, revitalization, self-confidence, learning, and maturation.[21] Not merely a functional tool, presence builds empathic engagement that benefits both client and practitioner.

RESPONDING TO THE STORY

Physician and anthropologist Paul Farmer notes that there are two ways of knowing and thus two ways of bearing witness. The first—to report the stoic suffering of the poor—is in every sense as genuine as another,

---

18. Salovey et al., *Emotional Intelligence*.

19. Spross, "Coaching and Suffering," 173–208.

20. Benner, *From Novice to Expert*, chapter 2.

21. Easter, "Construct Analysis," 362–77.

more freighted form of knowing. That is, it is true that members of any subjugated group do not expect to be received warmly even when they are sick or tired or wounded. They would not expect the sort of courtesy extended so effortlessly to the privileged. The silence of the poor is conditioned.[22]

As a professional, one is called to respond to the suffering of individuals and communities with a combination of professional skill and empathy. In the process, one is occasionally required to "bear witness" to the suffering of others. What is bearing witness or beholding suffering? Charon describes the task of the health-care worker as building true intersubjectivity with sick people. She writes, "Our narrative efforts toward ethicality and intersubjectivity enable us to not just *feel* on a patient's behalf but to commit acts of particularized and efficacious recognition that lead beyond empathy to the chance to restore power or control to those who have suffered."[23]

Restoring power to those who have been powerless is an essential aspect of dealing with those whose lives have been marked by fear. Thurman notes that those who live in fear of the dominant power group live in a fear that inhabits their physical body. Such fear is inherited from parent to child. Breaking the cycle of fear demands a radical shift in the way power is used by dominant groups who own power, privilege, or specialized knowledge, a group that includes helping professionals.

APPROPRIATING SUFFERING

Those who would bear witness, tell narratives on behalf of the suffering, or advocate for change must be imbued with a consciousness of the danger of appropriating suffering. Writers such as Farmer, James Orbinski, and others, who seek to put into words the suffering they have witnessed, do so with humility, recognizing it is in some sense their privilege that allows them to tell the story. The privilege carries the responsibility to not appropriate this story for false ends but to bear witness on behalf of the silenced or marginalized. The production of books, the need to raise funds for organizations, and the requirements of academic publishing challenge those whose use of those stories might result in unethical witness.

22. Farmer, *Pathologies of Power*, 25–28.
23. Charon, *Narrative Medicine*, 181.

The practice of regarding suffering can also degenerate into an emotive crater of liberal guilt. Liberal guilt creates communities of individuals who accept no responsibility to act but establish a moral superiority towards their focus. Critical understanding and theoretical sophistication is not a substitute for practice and action.

RE-PRESENTING SUFFERING

Having observed suffering, what does one do with the information or knowledge gained? Does knowledge demand action? Courses on poverty, for example, can present the information in a detached social scientific manner or can provide additional opportunities for students to imagine or experience the conditions of poverty. As an anthropology student in the Netherlands, I took a course on the history of Atlantic slavery. The students, who were mostly from former colonies and Caribbean islands, grew increasingly tense as the white, male instructor described the harsh realities of slave life. When challenged by the students, he shrugged his shoulders and responded, "I am just telling it the way it was."

Elizabeth Spelman asks important questions about the role of art in either representing or scavenging the suffering of those portrayed. When does it serve those suffering? Although some images have created huge shifts in public opinion, there is also the possibility that recurrent images in the media can create immunity and apathy instead of empathy. Documentary photography of the poor in New York City allows "viewers to convince themselves that they have gained the moral benefits of learning how the other half lives, without having to know such sufferers firsthand, without having any but their visual sense (and that at second hand) exposed to unspeakable living conditions."[24] Documentary photographers work in the tension of displaying "what is" and letting the conditions speak through the photograph. Shelby Lee Adams's photography of Appalachia depicts a reality that disturbs many. In a discussion of the increased images of violence in current times, Susan Sontag observes that people develop increased tolerance to these images. "Compassion is an unstable emotion. It needs to be translated into action, or it withers."[25]

24. Spelman, *Fruits of Sorrow*, 147.
25. Sontag, *Regarding the Pain of Others*, 101.

In suggesting that suffering demands a response from a practitioner, we need to examine the mechanisms that allow one to move from regarding to feeling to action. Moral principles of caring for the other are merely principles until they are somehow enacted. How does empathy activate previously taught moral principles? Goodman describes how empathy can trigger moral principles to help transform feelings into action and move one's moral concern out of the abstract and impersonal. Action can result from empathic distress as people attempt to reduce the negative arousal that they feel. In addition, she notes that empathy can move one out of narrow self-interest into a concern for others.[26]

Empathy can motivate action on behalf of others, or it can focus the individual inward. Martin Hoffman notes several self-destructing capacities of empathy, including egoistic drift. In this situation, self-focused role-taking can trigger a process in which one gets caught up in ruminating about one's own experiences and drifts out of the empathic mode.[27] Another self-destructing mechanism based on direct affect as well as empathic affect is habituation. If a person is exposed to another's distress repeatedly over time, habituation may occur, and the cumulative effect may be that the observer's empathic distress diminishes to the point of the person's becoming indifferent to the individual's suffering. Urban dwellers may become immune to the suffering of the homeless that line their daily travels to and from work.

Hoffman notes that empathy's limitations can be minimized when it is embedded in relevant moral principles. The cognitive dimension of moral principle helps give structure and stability to empathic affect. He argues that when one encounters another in distress, empathic distress is aroused, and one's empathically charged moral principles with their cognitive and affective components are activated. The empathic affect (principle-driven empathic distress) helps stabilize the empathic affect aroused by the victim (situation-driven empathic distress). Hoffman hypothesizes that abstract moral principles learned, for example, in lectures or sermons, lack motivating force. Empathy transforms moral principles into pro-social cognitions—thus giving them motivating force. The bond created between empathy and principle "creates a bond between them, which gives principle an affective charge."[28]

26. Goodman, *Promoting Diversity*, 138.
27. Hoffman, *Empathy and Moral Development*, 200.
28. Ibid., 239.

If the cycle of moving from regarding suffering to empathic connection to action requires both affective and cognitive components to keep this reaction balanced, it is essential that educators and mentors of students in professions provide both kinds of learning experiences. In the next section, we will examine the responses to suffering in the lives of certain individuals who regarded suffering and responded to it in creative ways. Empathy can activate the imagination, as well as provide an important motivator to create something new or to respond to social needs imaginatively.

CASE STUDIES

Concerning the capacity to feel the pain of others, James Orbinski writes, "In our choice to be with those who suffer, compassion leads not simply to pity but to solidarity. Solidarity implies a willingness to confront the causes and conditions of suffering that persist in destroying dignity, and to demand a minimum respect for human life. Solidarity also means recognizing the dignity and autonomy of others, and asserting the right of others to make choices about their own destiny. Humanitarianism is about the struggle to create the space to be fully human."[29] In the following short case studies, we will examine the biographies of individuals who used empathy to innovate and to bring dignity and awareness to conditions of suffering.

Joanna Macy (b. 1929)

In her memoir *Widening Circles*, Joanna Macy describes her childhood with an emotionally and times physically abusive father. The connection she formed in her youth with the Presbyterian Church provided her with a community that she identified with until the end of her studies at Wellesley College. Throughout her childhood, extended summers on her grandparent's farm near Buffalo brought her consolation from the emotionally contested space of her family's apartment in New York and instilled in her a deep love of nature.

Travels through India and Asia opened her understanding of a different form of spirituality and a more embodied compassion based on the interrelatedness of all being. Macy began studying Buddhist spirituality. Although she initially resisted the principle that all of life

---

29. Orbinski, *An Imperfect Offering*, 7–8.

is suffering (*dukkha*), she came to the realization that it was a profound truth. She writes, "All I knew was the story—the story of our living—was as much about suffering as it was about anything else. I could no more extricate life than take the eggs out of the batter, or lift the tapestry free from the warp on which it is woven."[30] Macy followed her husband in his career with the Peace Corps to Tunisia and then Nigeria, each time trying to find meaning and work in these new places.

She described attending a Quaker meeting where a man spoke about suffering in various places. Macy had a sudden insight of the potential for humans to be able to enter into the suffering of others, as she observes, "And then there was this inkling that in that entering something real could happen, something of enormous importance." It was a direction in which she hoped to be able to move.[31]

Macy became deeply involved in Buddhist practice, which culminated in a ritual that initiated her into the tradition. Along the way, she had visions and experiences that helped her see the unity in all reality. During one of these moments of insight, she notes, "A tenderness took hold—for myself, for the voices, for my people in this crazy time on Earth. It felt like abundance, embracing both our noble ideals and our daily absurdities; it felt like compassion."[32] Macy pursued advanced studies in systems theory and Buddhism at Syracuse University.

Although Macy moved outside of a strict adherence to the Christian faith of her youth, she never completely rejected that faith. She believed that there were connections between the faiths and a deeper truth that one could perceive. One Easter she noted that the message of Easter included death and the notion that "we are not separated or separable, that we belong to each other."[33]

Macy's conviction that the world was moving towards environmental catastrophe inspired her involvement in grassroots politics and nonviolent resistance movements. In 1979 she travelled to Sri Lanka to observe the work of Sarvodya Shramadana, a community development movement lead by a former teacher, Ari Ariyaratne.

Macy notes that one of her transformative moments was the awareness that one can be motivated by the desire to relieve the sufferings

30. Macy, *Widening Circles*, 100.

31. Ibid., 118.

32. Ibid., 106.

33. Ibid., 217.

of others. When one does not turn away from grief, a new connection emerges with the world and the people in it. Macy developed workshops where people could express both despair and re-engagement. In these workshops she allowed participants to voice their deepest feelings and shared with them a compassion that supports the interconnectedness with all life.[34] Through her own growth in empathy and her understanding of the need for others to do the same work, Macy has created educational processes that enable people to heal and to take up the cause of bearing witness in an enlightened way.

James P. Comer

James Comer, an African-American educator, was born in East Chicago, Indiana, in 1934. He was the son of a steel mill worker and a domestic. He received a BA from Indiana University, an MD from Howard University, and an MPH from the University of Michigan. Dr. Comer has long been associated with the Child Study Center at Yale University.[35] Comer was the second oldest of five children, whose parents were very involved in their schooling. In the book *Maggie's American Dream* (1989), Comer allows his mother's voice to describe their family life, accompanying it with his memories of growing up.

When Comer left home to attend Indiana University in Bloomington, he was overwhelmed by fear and alienation. He had used achievement to overcome obstacles in high school, but once at university he experienced overt discrimination at the university and in the town itself. Many black students dropped out, not because they were inadequately prepared for college, but because they "were defeated by the social situation."[36] Comer was accepted into Indiana Medical School, but he decided instead to attend the predominantly black Howard University. Comer trained in child psychiatry, and his contact with patients shaped his later educational platform. He observed that before meeting some of his clients he thought that hard work brought success, but he realized that society was preventing many people from attaining success. While moonlighting in a general practice and considering his future, Comer realized, "Nothing in my medical bag was going to solve the problems I saw around me—

34. Macy, *Coming Back to Life*, 212.
35. Comer, *What I Learned in School*.
36. Comer, *Beyond Black and White*, 35.

the roaches, the poverty, the depression."[37] He returned to Washington in 1961 to spend two years working for the U.S. Public Health Service. He volunteered at Hospitality House, a shelter for women and children. His interest was preventive psychiatry, so he completed his MPH and then did a two-year residency at Yale, followed by a fellowship in child psychiatry.

While he was sorting out his own need to achieve, Comer was also trying to understand why society interpreted black behavior in unflattering light. He noticed that black people's inability to achieve was often attributed to laziness rather than to structural obstacles.

While counseling a young patient named Walter, Comer realized that his own success could be attributed to factors that were outside his direct control, such as his family and community. Working with such complex cases and seeing how limited his patients' chances of success were, Comer realized that education was a key factor. He believed that educators tend to blame the children and their parents for a school's failure, while as a society we have failed to meet the basic needs of people. The school system was only a by-product of the larger failure.

One of Comer's main concerns was the improvement of the academic performance of children from low-income or minority backgrounds. He believed one cannot focus on the child and family while ignoring the other variables that affect achievement and learning. He acknowledged the stressful conditions under which many students live, which prevent them from learning to socialize and play in the way schools expect them to. This, in turn, interferes with their learning. Comer designed a proposal, later called the Comer method, to address this problem. The method created a governance and management team within each school, which was led by the principal and made up of elected teacher and parent representatives and a mental-health worker from Yale Child Study Center. The project focused on self-esteem and social-skills development. Comer writes, "It was my own family experience, our knowledge of child development, and our experience in the first five years of the project that led us to focus on social development and social skills."[38]

The Comer method has since spread throughout the country. From its beginning at two elementary schools in New Haven in 1967, the program showed radical success in reading and math levels, attendance,

37. Comer, *Maggie's American Dream*, 190.
38. Ibid., 217.

and improved behavior. In 1990 the Rockefeller Foundation announced that it would spend five years and fifteen million dollars adopting the program in the United States. Comer continues to work and advocate for educational systems, teachers, and families who address the systemic issues that defeat certain students.

Florence Wald (1917–2008)

Florence Wald was born in New York City and graduated from Mount Holyoke College in 1938. She completed a graduate degree in nursing at Yale University in 1941 and an MS at Yale Graduate School in 1956. Her professional experience included work as a staff nurse for a visiting nurse service, research assistant at the College of Physicians and Surgeons, and instructor at Rutgers University School of Nursing. In 1957 she was appointed to the Yale School of Nursing where she served as professor, researcher, and dean.

A meeting with Cicely Saunders, founder of St. Christopher's Hospice in England (established 1965), led to a growing friendship between the two women and planted the idea for the development of a hospice in the United States. Wald began studying dying patients and their families, and her interdisciplinary team organized care for these families and met regularly to discuss their findings. The study helped shape the mission and guiding principles for the founding of Hospice Inc. in the New Haven area. Wald served on the Board of Directors and on the planning staff until she resigned in 1975. Her husband Henry served on the Board until 1977 and chaired the Building and Site Committee. Hospice Inc. began planning for a permanent site and worked on design, funds, policies, and staff for that building. The home care program began seeing patients in 1974. The inpatient program began in 1979 in the building in Branford, Connecticut, renamed Connecticut Hospice Inc.

The "Nurse's Study of Care for Dying Patients" gathered an interdisciplinary team to discuss the findings. Patients in the study who represented a variety of ethnic backgrounds and social class were studied in different settings, including their homes, a nursing home, a clinic, and hospital wards. Practitioners participating in the study were clearly influenced by the work of Dr. Elisabeth Kübler-Ross in the late 1960s, in particular the five stages of dying that she describes in her book *On Death and Dying*. Using a diary technique, the nurses recorded relevant details about each patient's physical or emotional condition, as well as observations of the family members. They noticed that patients improved at unexpected times and sometimes declined unexpectedly in ways that seemed to be more related to other events or relationships than to disease.

Wald included the patients' environments as one of the factors that seemed to influence the course of their dying. She observes, "I think the effect of the environment, especially the degree of independence that the patient can have and his ability to have a role as a human being seems to correlate with both psychological symptoms and physical symptoms."[39] She believed it was important to determine how illness affected family dynamics. She did an assessment on intake and then also during the process, since many changes took place in the patient or in the family that were sometimes surprising to the researchers. Wald noted that healthcare practitioners could have an influence on the patient. She felt that nurses sometimes gave ambiguous messages to the patient that resulted in the patient not knowing how to act. One patient commented one day that with her family lined up beside her bed, it looked as if they were at a funeral parlor. When the nurses took up that cue and behaved less as if she were a dying patient, her condition improved.[40]

Wald was concerned that her team had not really observed the stage that Kübler-Ross described as "acceptance." The study group felt that additional research should include the financial situation of the family, pain control, the role of anxiety and anti-depressants, and the function of hope. As the group continued to meet and deal with the complexities of the dying process and bereavement among families, the intensity of the work at times affected the staff who participated. One worker noted that Wald's commitment, overwork, and anxiety made her feel guilty for not doing enough. The worker told Wald, "I know you don't intend it, but I'm saying that's the way [it is]—so that if I were to get sick the night before our conference, I would say—Oh my God, I can't because there is Florence working away, you know, I must come in."[41]

At a meeting of the interdisciplinary group (October 29, 1970), Wald expressed her continuing commitment caring for the dying patient and his or her family. She noted that she felt a deep responsibility to meet the

---

39. Wald, "Proceedings of a Conference," 40.

40. Ibid.

41. Wald, "Unidentified Group Member" in Notebooks (Vol. 8, June 1970), Yale Archives.

needs of those faced with the end of life. This care included the physical needs of the patient, so that "the person can be free to see the meaning of his total life despite his incapacity, as well as his relationship to other people. Then perhaps he can think of himself as indestructible in terms of the spirit that is within him, and is and will be in other people."[42]

Wald observed the suffering of patients and their families in their end-of-life situations. The longer-term study allowed certain themes to emerge that enabled her to propose better care for individuals in home, hospital, or hospice settings. She also realized that professionals needed to be schooled in caring for the dying patient and the family to provide the basis for honest and meaningful communication.

An interdisciplinary team was well suited to meet the complex physical, emotional, and spiritual needs of the patient. Pain control was an essential part of that care. In addition, the environment of care was important, and the architecture of the proposed hospice in Connecticut became the focus of much study. All these aspects have become so much a part of hospice and palliative care philosophy that it is easy to forget that a few decades ago, such ideas were novel and were even resisted by medical caregivers. Wald's work in hospice and later in prisons derived from empathy for a population whose needs were unmet.

Jean Vanier (b. 1928)

Jean Vanier bought a house in 1964 in a village north of Paris and lived there with three disabled adults. He was motivated by the desire to do good, but he did not realize that "those people would 'do good' to him."[43] From this beginning grew the community named L'Arche, which became a worldwide movement based on respect for the differently abled. Son of a devout mother and a respected lawyer and WWI veteran, Jean Vanier was born in Geneva, where his father was a military advisor to the Canadian delegation at the League of Nations. His father later became the Governor General of Canada. Jean chose a career in the navy by joining the Royal Naval College at Dartmouth.[44]

While on leave in Paris in 1945, Vanier was deeply affected when he saw survivors of four concentration camps arrive at the station.

---

42. Wald, Group No. 1659, Series V, Box 27, Folder No. 71, Yale Archives.

43. Spink, *The Miracle*, 1.

44. Ibid., 19.

Other influences included a visit with his father to Lourdes and a visit to Friendship House in Harlem. After serving eight years in the navy, he wondered if he had a vocation to be a priest. His mother introduced him to a French Dominican priest, Father Thomas Phillippe, who had started a community outside Paris called Living Water. The priest became an important mentor to the former navy officer. Vanier supported the notion of filiation as a way of spiritual formation, as opposed to studying in universities with professional educators. While in Paris, he wrote a doctoral thesis on Aristotle. After a year of teaching ethics at the University of Toronto, Vanier returned to France at the suggestion of his mentor that he might involve himself in ministry to the disabled.

Vanier established a home in Trosly-Breuil and invited three disabled men to live with him. Vanier quickly realized that he was not there to help them, but to learn to listen. By living with the two remaining men (one had to be sent back to an institution), Vanier realized "not only immense pain but also beauty and gentleness, a capacity for communion and tenderness."[45] There were a variety of influences on Vanier's valuing of the poor: in particular, his contact with the Little Sisters and Brothers of Jesus in Montreal, and Dorothy Day's paper *The Catholic Worker*. He felt that his work needed to focus on those with intellectual disabilities.[46]

The work spread as volunteers arrived to work in France or to open new communities around the world. The work at L'Arche emphasized living with rather than just experiencing. This led the volunteer workers to experience healing. As Spinks describes it, "In some mysterious way a reciprocal healing took place and at its most profound level it was possibly that healing which confirmed people in L'Arche."[47] Vanier's work continues today around the world in communities where the needs of the differently abled had previously been ignored.

Dorothy Day (1897–1980)

Dorothy Day was born in New York City in 1897, the third child of John Day, a journalist, and Grace Day, a homemaker. The family moved from New York to San Francisco to Chicago. Day attended university at the University of Illinois (Urbana). She did not complete her university edu-

---

45. Ibid., 64.
46. Ibid.
47. Ibid., 206.

cation, but instead moved to New York to work as a journalist. Biographer Robert Coles notes that she became part of the radical Greenwich Village scene, where she honed "a passionate sense of justice."[48] The next years were marked by protest, imprisonment, travel, and a succession of failed relationships. When a novel she had written was turned into a screenplay, she used the proceeds to purchase a cottage on Staten Island. Day gave birth to a daughter, Tara. She separated shortly after from her common-law husband, who was not interested in fatherhood or in Day's growing interest in the Catholic Church. Living in New York with her young child, Day was surrounded by the human suffering caused by the Depression. The indifference of social institutions like the church to the suffering of those around affected her deeply.

In university Day had joined the socialist party. Her readings and contacts at the time made it seem as if religion was in conflict with social conditions of poverty, since religion preached meekness and joy. She could not understand why energy was spent in attempting to remedy social conditions, instead of trying to eliminate injustice. Moving back to New York, she spent days exploring the city and neighborhoods and writing for a socialist paper. During this time she experienced what she described as the long loneliness—a time when she was in the big city with no friends, no one to talk to, and surrounded by silence in the noise of the city. She was appalled by the poverty she saw around her, but she also felt a call to live in the middle of these conditions. She felt that if she didn't, she would never be freed from the burden of loneliness.

While picketing the White House with a group of suffragists, Day was jailed with the others who engaged in a hunger strike. The experience crushed her in its misery; she observed that it was one thing to understand suffering theoretically, but quite another to experience it firsthand. A few years later she was again arrested, and her experience in jail made her feel that she was sharing the life of the poorest. To counter the long loneliness, Day believed that people should find ways to live in community.

Her thoughts on community also urged the involvement of citizens in local politics. She argued, "We would like to see more small communities organizing themselves, people talking with people, people *caring* for people, people coming together in order to make known what they

48. Coles, *Dorothy Day*, 3.

believe and what they would like their nation to do. Apathy, like sloth, is a sin."[49]

Day described her life as being divided into two parts. She describes the first twenty-five years as the floundering years, which were followed by her conversion to Catholicism and work with the Catholic Worker movement.[50]

Day's meeting with activist Peter Maurin set the course for the next part of her life, as they became collaborators on the newspaper *The Catholic Worker* and worked to establish houses of hospitality to provide charity for those in need. She reflected on her own interest in questions of justice: "He [God] put us here to *ask,* to try to find out the best way possible to live with our neighbors. Of course you can go through life not asking, and that's the tragedy: so many lives lived in moral blindness."[51]

Day documents the history of the Catholic Worker in her book *Loaves and Fishes.* She also describes the communitarian farms and the theory of voluntary poverty. For Day, poverty was an important way to live. She writes, "The act and spirit of giving are the best counter to the evil forces in the world today, and giving liberates the individual not only spiritually but materially."[52]

The network of hospitality houses and farms founded by Day and Maurin continue in the United States and Canada, as well as in other countries. Dorothy Day saw the suffering of workers and unemployed people and was moved to provide bread and care for those people. Her empathy brought her to bear witness on behalf of the poor through the workers' houses and the newsletter. Her work derived from a deeply spiritual and personal place that gave her courage to protest publicly and to live in discomfort herself.

CONCLUSION

There are many others who have stood with the suffering and taken the opportunity to bear witness on their behalf. Empathy and personal experience of suffering helped these individuals to be agents of change, working for justice. None of these individuals would claim to be extraor-

49. Coles, *Dorothy Day,* 107–8.

50. Day, *Long Loneliness,* 21.

51. Ibid., 24.

52. Day, *Loaves and Fishes,* 86.

dinary; rather, they were moved by their own experiences of suffering to witness on behalf of others and to act for change. Empathy can be empowering to those who seek to use their professional skills to work for justice. In the next chapter, we will identify the skills associated with empathy and look at how one can improve the empathic ability.

QUESTIONS FOR FURTHER DISCUSSION

1. What are the components of a story or narrative?

2. Do you have family stories of sickness? Interview one of your relatives or friends about their experience.

3. Read an illness narrative. Compare the story to Arthur Frank's description of illness narratives.

4. Watch a film that deals with an illness story. Summarize the plot. How did family or friends react to the patient? What, from your point of view, was helpful?

5. Research artists who work with themes of suffering and witness. What do they hope to accomplish through art?

6. This chapter has presented several case studies of individuals who responded to suffering in creative ways. Find another individual who is not mentioned here. Read his or her biography. What were important factors in their lives that helped them to see the suffering of others, and what did they do to respond to it?

5

Improving the Empathic Ability

AS A STUDENT IN my final weeks of nursing school, I returned to the nurses' residence after an absence of several days. I had attended the funeral of my older brother, who had died unexpectedly. My clinical group was sent to the morgue to learn care of the body after death. I observed the clinical instructor bathe the patient, stabilize the jaw, pack the body with cotton, and wrap the body in a shroud, to make it ready to be picked up by the funeral director. That this learning experience might be too uncomfortable after my brother's sudden death did not seem to cross the instructor's mind—and I would not have asked for an exception. If the situation was a test of my ability to hold steady as a detached professional, then I was determined to pass the test.

The cold basement, the dead body, the caps and polyester-garbed students seemed like a bad dream. The only way to prove that I was up to the task was to detach emotionally and make joking asides to my fellow students. Such emotional detachment seemed to be an essential skill for a student nurse in training. Although caring was encouraged, emotional involvement interfered with professional expectations. The incident was not discussed in the conference afterward. The ethical modeling was clear and powerful—duty trumped feelings. The notion of self-care had not yet emerged as part of the professional conversation.

Reflecting on this incident many decades later, it seems to me that a pedagogical opportunity had been missed. Kübler-Ross's work *On Death and Dying* had been published a few years earlier, but her ideas about death were just beginning to filter into small-town hospitals. I missed an opportunity to speak up and share my experience with my clinical group and the instructor. Instead, I learned how detach in the professional setting and modeled this to my fellow students. The clinical instructor lost an opportunity to model empathy and to discuss the connections between observing suffering in professional practice and experiencing suffering personally. Ignoring the cumulative effect of extended exposure to suffering by helping professionals can have negative effects on their personal and professional lives. When the suffering self finds expression through reflection and discussion, it can provide a point of deep connection with others. When suppressed, the suffering self experiences disconnection and an inability to experience empathy.

One of the tasks of professional education is to establish clear boundaries between the care of a client and the care of the professional. The fear of emotional engagement is tied to the threat of emotional overload. The challenge for a professional is not only to engage in an authentic way but also to have boundaries in place that allow the emotion to strengthen the technical sides of the work, not undermine them. In addition, in many settings the relationship between client and practitioner is mediated by technology that can in some cases facilitate the relationship (telemedicine, distance education, web-enabled communication, and email), and in other cases distract from the relationship (practitioners who focus solely on the evidence of monitors and instruments and make no contact with the patient).

FORMING THE EMPATHIC QUALITIES
OF AN IDEAL PRACTITIONER

Curriculum for the helping professions includes elements of explicit, implicit, null, and hidden curriculum. Curriculum is rarely static—schools regularly undergo revisions in an attempt to keep the content current and related to the mission and vision statement of the school. Professional formation occurs in classroom, internships, practica, service learning, interaction with peers, and information networks outside of the academy. Not only the content, but the method and the culture of the professional school instruct the student in professional practice. Many professional schools resist changing instructional methodology despite pressures to accommodate adaptive versus technical ways of knowing. Rather than memorizing blocks of content, professionals increasingly need skills such as information seeking and critical analysis, as well as contextualizing knowledge and experience.

As we have seen in chapter 1, professional schools create boundaries by means of specialized knowledge and standards of practice. Accreditation for professional schools depends on standards set by an external body that monitors the quality of education.[1] The accreditation process for professional schools evaluates the overall effectiveness of individual schools in forming professionals with desired knowledge, skills, and attitudes. Implicit values supported through accreditation may include either a commitment to serve underserved populations or, by contrast, helping an individual with no reference to larger social issues. Public opinion and media coverage regularly target the training of professionals and occasionally suggest that the professional education is inadequate or that new skills are needed.[2] Change is often slow in such programs, as instructors replicate the way they were taught rather than experimenting with pedagogical innovation. And such innovation is not always valued and rewarded by the institutions in which professionals are educated.

Most professional schools likely agree that empathy is important, but they might have different ways to teach or sustain empathy throughout their programs. Some professions require some evidence of a predisposition to empathy in a candidate prior to admission (as expressed in a personal statement or volunteer commitments), whereas other programs aim to provide or supplement empathic skills during the education. Because there is some confusion as to whether empathy is an inherent personality characteristic or whether it can be taught, it is difficult for educational programs to specifically identify where the curriculum supports empathic engagement or to demonstrate how this learning can be measured. The rhetoric of empathy as a desirable trait is often disconnected from pedagogical specificity. In addition, the essentializing discourse of each profession hinders inter-professional debate. Not only are there very different understandings of what empathy consists of, and how it might be taught, but also each profession may claim a different language to describe what empathy means. The danger of such an isolated discussion is that if the language is only intelligible to insiders to the profession, the debate remains internal. The esoteric nature of professional language makes it difficult to communicate with other professions or to convince others that the work is important to the organization as a whole.[3]

1. Insitute of Medicine, *Nation's Compelling Interest*, 127.

2. Wallace, "Multicultural Critical Theory"; Chen, "Do You Have the Right Stuff?"

3. Holmes and Gastaldo, "Rhizomatic Thought in Nursing." *Nursing Philosophy* 5 (2004): 258–67.

Salovey classifies empathy as an aspect of emotional intelligence that includes such skills as emotional appraisal and expression of emotion, regulation of emotions, and utilization of emotions.[4] Empathy can be seen as a motivator for altruistic behavior.[5] Empathy may include the ability to understand another's point of view, identify accurately another's emotions, experience the same or other emotions in response, and communicate or act on this internal experience. Salovey describes stages of empathic connection that include the perception "as if" one were the other, feeling with another, and acting on the feeling. A professional may recognize the "as if" stage and might also feel with the person, but then may resist acting on those feelings.

Although many would agree that empathy could be enhanced by education, there may not be agreement on the importance of empathic abilities for professionals. Could a technically proficient student be failed for exhibiting an empathy deficit? Throughout history emotions have generally been viewed with skepticism and associated with weakness and vulnerability. The Stoics of ancient Greece, for example, saw emotion as an unreliable source of wisdom, whereas the late-eighteenth- to early-nineteenth-century Romantics favored emotion as a valuable source of insight.[6]

In a professional context it is considered appropriate to rejoice with one who rejoices, but it is more troubling to weep with those who weep (Rom 12:15). Having the ability to be engaged in the empathic process, that is, to stand in the "as if" situation, feel the emotions, and act on them, depends on the individual's own understanding of the nature of suffering.

Farrell and Muscari argue that an empathic individual risks that "the relationship will evoke strong feelings, especially if the professional has experienced the same situation that is being described."[7] For example, students who are breast cancer survivors, or who have experienced family struggles with homelessness, addictions, or chronic illness, may be challenged when caring for patients in similar situations. Professional or therapeutic empathy is a complex skill that should not be confused with simply being kind or affectively engaged. Professional training programs

4. Salovey et al., *Emotional Intelligence*, 60.

5. Batson, "Prosocial Motivation," 65–122.

6. Salovey et al., *Emotional Intelligence*, 62.

7. Farrell and Muscari, "Empathy," 65–73.

can help students learn the boundaries of empathic engagement, free of manipulation or distortion of the professional relationship, and also free of empathic overload.

If professional education can enhance empathy, does empathy develop in stages or in sudden transformative moments of increased self-understanding? Some envision the empathetic process as including a biological state whereby individuals experience their own bodily actions, grow increasingly attuned to their own responses and feelings, and then become aware of the other. Regardless of the exact steps, the information is filtered through a lens that involves the personal first (evaluation of one's response) and then allows one to enter into the "as if" of the other.

A description of empathic engagement involving stages has much in common with many descriptions of faith formation or faith development theory that have roots in the development psychology of the twentieth century. Students' responses to the suffering of others and their degree of self-awareness will have different starting places. Some need help managing overwhelming feelings of empathy, whereas others need to access the affective domain. Mentoring is essential in helping to learn to manage the affective overload or the cognitive dissonance that witnessing suffering can trigger.

EDUCATION FOR EMPATHY—CHANGING TYPES OF LEARNING AND TEACHING

Higher-education programs are increasingly encouraging reflective or contemplative thinking to enhance critical thinking and empathic ability. A traditional curriculum focused on obtaining a body of knowledge, whereas current educators recognize that the body of knowledge is always changing and students need to have skills in obtaining, updating, and integrating this constantly shifting knowledge base. Although critical thinking is generally valued more highly than rote memorization, it is rarely enough. Students need opportunities to apply theories in order to practice focusing on individual differences in context. This process depends on direct engagement with individuals and communities rather than the comfortable detachment that academic inquiry has often supported.

Debates about the essential core (whether art or science) of a professional training will continue to support or undermine new initiatives in curriculum. Teachers in professional schools have many ways to subvert a curriculum that does not reflect their own priorities; conversely, teachers can bring a high degree of creativity to a curriculum that has long ago lost touch with professional realities. Innovations in the professional curriculum may include changes in courses (ethics), modes of teaching (teacher- vs. learner-centered), emphases (science vs. humanities), ways of learning (problem-based learning versus lecture), collaborative learning (small group exercises), service learning, and increased exposure over time to clients. In search of empathic candidates, therefore, professional schools can either scrutinize students on admission, provide empathic training during the course of education, work to help students retain capacities they already have, or use lifelong learning programs to emphasize the continued importance of empathy over the course of a career. Documenting and evaluating the effectiveness of empathy-focused education will continue to challenge the assessment aspects of teaching.

QUALITIES RELATED TO AN EMPATHIC PRACTITIONER

Professional schools identify characteristics of ideal graduates armed with the skills, knowledge, and attitudes obtained during their education. Some of these skills, knowledge, and attitudes may not explicitly be called empathy but may be closely or implictly associated with the ideal of an empathic practitioner. In the next section we will examine some of those qualities that are elements of professional empathy in order to broaden our understanding of what empathy entails.

JUSTICE—WORKING FOR RIGHT RELATIONS

Educating for justice creates a critical understanding of the student's privilege while developing insight into the complex realities of the other. Transformative learning courses with a focus on justice often begin with self-location as the beginning of critical reflection on attitudes to race, ethnicity, religion, class, educational background, and networks of privilege. This transformative learning task precedes the identification of structural problems and oppressive patterns in larger relationships. In addition, such self-awareness is essential to the ability to identify invisible privilege, to effectively forge partnerships between people and organizations, and to monitor the empathic response to the self and to the other, as described above.

Self-awareness is one aspect of a skill or intelligence that is related to empathy. This awareness is not a version of professional narcissism, but rather an honest reflection on one's complicity with conditions of inequity and lack of empathy. Clinical and practical experiences do not always expand students' understanding of the other; students who deal with disadvantaged populations in their training do not necessarily emerge with greater empathy. Indeed, stereotypes can be reinforced and left unchallenged. Exposure to conditions of poverty that are not accompanied with skills in social analysis can leave students frustrated by empathic overload that offers no guidance on action and follow-up.

An Australian study of nursing practice with patients of non-English-speaking background took place in a large metropolitan hospital. The nurses who participated in the study were required to reflect on their practice, to see their own constructions of white and Western notions of individual and family that actually harmed their patients. Over time, the nurses had to be taught to see the intersection of gender, race, and ethnicity, because their own privilege made these interconnections invisible to them. Exclusionary practices were not only the result of the nurses' actions, but also of "broader institutional and government policies that shape and constrain nursing practice."[8] The article describing this study concludes with the recommendation that nurses need to establish negotiated partnerships "with the stakeholders of health care to make the rhetoric of multiculturalism in mainstream health care a reality."[9]

In creating a transformative awareness, Anne Curry-Stevens describes the following process: students become aware of oppression; see it as structural, enduring, and pervasive; locate themselves as oppressed; locate themselves as privileged; understand the benefits that flow from privilege; and understand themselves as implicated in the oppression of others. The final step allows students to declare intentions for future action.[10] Her study of a group of community educators indicates that in different contexts people will experience degrees of either privilege or oppression, and a transformative process needs to take those into account.

Working towards right relations thus assumes a degree of self-awareness in relation to others. Teaching the reflective skills to monitor

8. Blackford, "Cultural Frameworks," 238.

9. Ibid., 242.

10. Curry-Stevens, "New Forms of Transformative Education," 33–58.

one's motivations for professional helping is an essential skill for those who choose to work for justice. Such reflection demands the ability to critically examine one's deepest motivations during times of great dedication and times of deep fatigue.[11] Building on such reflective skills and self-awareness, professional education can supplement cognitive knowledge with skills in advocacy, education, and transformative learning to practitioners that prepare them to work at the individual and structural level to eliminate disparities in education, health, and housing.

The motivation behind helping others or working towards right relations must be carefully scrutinized so that the professional works out of care rather than the desire to control. Thomas R. Kelly notes that it is important to ask if we want to help people because we feel sorry for them or because we genuinely love them. He noted that the world needs "something deeper than pity; it needs love."[12] Such idealism may be out of touch with the learning culture of many professional schools; however, engaging students in the possibility of change and hope can create conditions for optimism that result in more relational professional care. Professional resilience and longevity depend on such reflective abilities.

The starting point or mission of any professional program sets the tone for the engagement of students and the potential enhancement of empathy. While advocating for prophetic teachers, David Purpel claims that teachers must start with a focus on the actual challenges that people face, such as poverty, war, hunger, and injustice. Connecting to realities of people's lives facilitates new purpose for teaching. He writes, "I believe, however, that there are strong connections and it is these connections which give educators purpose and enable us to see ourselves as having prophetic responsibilities."[13]

CULTURAL COMPETENCE—UNDERSTANDING OTHERNESS AND READING DIFFERENCE

Many professional schools support cultural competence as a learning outcome. Students will serve a diverse client population—a diversity that is often not yet evident in either the faculty or student population. Competencies in intercultural, multicultural, or cross-cultural skills may

---

11. Thurman, "Mysticism and Social Action," 14–35.

12. Kelly, *Testament of Devotion*, 77.

13. Purpel, *Moral and Spiritual Crisis in Education*, 106.

also be supported by accrediting organizations. Desired nursing competencies, for example, include the skills, knowledge, and attitudes that allow one to provide care to diverse populations and to practice across the illness continuum, across the lifespan, and in collaboration with a variety of professionals. Understanding difference can include understanding ethnic and racial diversity, socioeconomic diversity, rural or urban diversity, as well as all the factors that cause migrations, movement, and displacement of people from their cultural homes. In medicine, diversity has been taught by means of a cultural competency approach (focusing on broad groupings of language and customs), a communication skills approach (focusing on individual descriptions using the client's own language), or a combination of the two. However, only eight percent of medical schools offer a separate course to address such issues, and most diversity-oriented teaching is restricted to the preclinical years. The hidden and unintended curriculum of professional schools supports the dominant culture.[14] In order to untangle the complex web of white privilege, faculties need to make a long-term commitment to radically reconsider how their school's curriculum, culture, and other practices (interviewing candidates, for example) supports the dominant culture.

Although understanding diversities is often included in the learning outcomes of professional education, the exact nature of this desired ability to deal with diversity is sometimes unclear. What specific skills, knowledge, and attitudes are students expected to obtain? Diversity and difference encompass the various expressions of culture, language, religion, and social customs that are influenced by gender, education, class, and other factors. A respect for diversities includes not only an understanding of things shared by a culture or faith group but also a respect for individual divergence from those group traits. Cognitive acceptance of diversity might not include an empathic or relational engagement with diversity. For a professional, recognizing or accepting diversity may go no further than checking off a box concerning a patient's ethnic or racial identity or denominational affiliation on an admission chart. The challenge remains for students to gain a deeper understanding of the overlapping aspects of gender, race, class, ethnicity and the ways that these are supported or constrained by their education and the organizations in which they work.

---

14. Institute of Medicine, *Nation's Compelling Interest*, 374.

Practitioners in an increasingly diverse society require complex skills to deal with diversity. They must not only understand one ethnic or cultural group, but also realize the transformations and complexities within each, depending on situation, immigration, marriage outside the group, location or relocation from urban to rural or rural to urban. As long as faculties and student populations are largely representative of dominant culture, how can meaningful understanding of diversity occur? If student populations are further fragmented into subgroups of like kind and interaction is limited between other groups, learning about diversity and difference will be a challenge.

Dynamic cultural pluralism encourages individuals to move beyond their initial subgroups to form communities of interest based on shared values. The process is dynamic and reflects changing concerns or issues that would enhance the group's mutual interest. Balancing the interests of the individual and the group is the challenge in this dynamic and shifting cultural system. Society would make room for competing ways of life without declaring any particular one as best. Education plays an important role in giving students tools for understanding diversities.[15]

Pluralism of value systems need not come at the expense of social cohesion. However, education systems must prepare individuals to acquire the skills, knowledge, and moral disposition to function autonomously in society. Education must teach the value of diversity and the importance of individual commitment to shared values in society.[16] Cultural pluralism invites individuals to move beyond their initial subgroups to form communities of interest groups. The balance between the freedom of individual autonomy and the preservation of ethnic heritage is a tension that individuals and communities negotiate. Learning bicultural values of both the ethnic group of origin and the dominant culture may allow some students to function in both without being forced to choose one over the other. Singh notes that at times these two cultures will conflict with each other. A dialogical process of working out these conflicts will be instructive for all. Professional students bring their own cultures of origin to the classroom and continue to negotiate understandings of diversities both in the classroom and in practice settings.

Contemporary professional education requires an adaptation to an environment that is pluricultural, complex, and almost limitless.

15. Singh, "Cultural Pluralism," 71.

16. Ibid., 78.

Migration and political pressures have created a situation of unprecedented cultural diversity. To meet the challenges of these complex diversities, education must face a new challenge—to protect personal identity and difference and support social integration.

Democracy itself must be rebuilt on the basis of difference. Josep Rovira argues that education must respond to this almost limitless increase in complexity. New ways of learning must help individuals make genuine contact with diverse others. Intercultural education seeks to work towards understanding between the individual's own culture and that with which he or she is making contact through dialogue that increases understanding beyond mere co-existence. Dialogue is necessary because contact challenges co-existence and collective survival.[17]

The helping professions will address increasing complexity and diversity. The ability to imagine diversities and difference beyond our personal experience requires a well-developed degree of empathic ability. Curriculum content, pedagogy, and contextual experience of difference will be essential to the helping professionals who serve not only clients like themselves but who increasingly welcome the world into waiting rooms, classrooms, and faith communities. This encounter with difference has the potential to energize the practice of helping professionals who learn to delight in the infinite variety of humanity even as they recognize the commonality of human experience in the form of suffering and hope.

SPIRITUALITY—RESPECTING BELIEF

Although most professional students are advised to keep their personal beliefs separate as much as possible from practice, there are times when the development of a professional persona is inextricably linked with core beliefs and values. How one understands the role of suffering and the place of hope are crucial when dealing with clients who experience hardship and challenge. A recent newspaper article described how a group of males who had recently been laid off from their jobs suffered a high incidence of heart attacks. How can one understand the connections between the body and the spirit, or grief and illness, without a deeper understanding of the role of belief, faith, joy, hope, and spiritual values on the body, as well as gender and cultural expectations? How

---

17. Ibid., 89.

can students with deep spiritual commitments learn to be tolerant and accepting in the workplace of different belief systems? How can students who devalue the spiritual realm cultivate appreciation for those who hold different beliefs? Spiritual commitments can be a source of spiritual self-care for the professional, but they require a clear understanding of the boundaries of personal belief and the imposition of such beliefs on clients.

Is there a way to gain an appreciation for spiritual values that incorporates rather than erases student spirituality? Does the professional curriculum have a place for students to discuss ultimate values and spiritual formation? Models of spiritual development have described different stages of individual awareness and ability to articulate personal values.[18] In addition, individual development has also been described as the ability to articulate empathic caring for another.[19] The discussions of values, ethics, change, and empathy have an important place in a professional curriculum.

The process of professional education may transform the ultimate beliefs of students. This may involve a loss of previously held worldview or adaptation or adoption of a totally new one. The starting place of each student will be different depending on life experiences and a host of other factors. In order to teach students to respect the beliefs of clients, it seems logical that professional schools should attempt to respect the students' beliefs first. Discussions of faith that are based in respect can enhance understanding of the other and prepare practitioners to extend empathy towards those who hold very different beliefs. Rather than checking off a box on a admissions form, students can learn to ask themselves how they practice their faith, what it means to them, if they share this view with their family, and how it prepares them for their current experience.

Exposure to other faiths or an examination of faith-development theory can be a useful framework for practitioners who will encounter issues of faith, spirituality, hope, despair, and death in the course of their practice.[20] Being comfortable with such topics may provide a more grounded ability to empathize. In addition, an understanding

18. Sperry, *Spirituality in Clinical Practice*.

19. Aldridge, *Spirituality, Healing and Medicine*.

20. Fowler, *Stages of Faith*.

of spirituality can support the role of self-care and reflection in the professional's career.

Our lives and choices are guided by ultimate values and worldviews. These values are integrated into our professional lives. As a professional skill, one might be able to identify one's own beliefs, contradictions, and changes in belief over time. In addition, helping professionals need the ability to understand, respect, or appreciate the beliefs, values, and points of view of the client or community. The ideal of a detached practitioner suggests that one can step away from core beliefs to a professional presence that is unaffected by core beliefs and values. Such detachment not only creates an inauthentic presence for the client but also leaves students defenseless when a situation arises that threatens their basic beliefs.

Arthur Chickering observes that higher education has paid little attention to the student's inner development, including values and beliefs, emotional maturity, moral development, spirituality, and self-understanding. Self-understanding through reflection is essential to understanding others. In his estimation, academic culture has encouraged people to live fragmented and inauthentic lives "in which we act as if we were not spiritual beings or as if our spiritual side were irrelevant to our vocation or work."[21]

How can one define spirituality in an inclusive way that fits the professional preparation of diverse types of helping professionals? Spirituality may describe a personal commitment to a process of inner development that engages us in our totality including phrases like a way of life; a contemplative attitude; a search for ultimate meaning, direction and belonging; and a commitment to growth as a lifelong goal. Although many professions have chosen science as their frame of reference, it presents limitations in understanding. Science is based on description of external observable facts, and the language of science does not work well with inner experiences. Higher education has increasingly relied on a mode of thinking that Palmer describes as objectivism and Chickering describes as rational empiricism, which "delegitimizes active public discussion of issues of purpose and meaning, authenticity and identity, spirituality and spiritual growth."[22]

21. Chickering et al., *Encouraging Authenticity*, x.
22. Ibid., 8–30.

Spirituality can describe a wide variety of skills, including dialogue, respect, and intuitive learning.[23] The learning process itself can be seen as a spiritual journey as individuals learn to question their presumptions, accept challenges to beliefs, and reframe their values. Ultimate spiritual values include reflecting on one's own values and purpose, as well as the need to care and be concerned for others. Rather than separate beliefs and values from their studies, students can be encouraged to reflect on their learning and consider how their initial sense of vocation changes as they progress from beginner to graduating practitioner.

One way to open discussions related to faith can be to examine theories of faith development that provide models for reflection about human change and growth on the spiritual level. Whether this development is seen as stages or spirals, the notion of spiritual unfolding challenges those who wish to have a more comprehensive view of the spiritual life over the life span and not merely a snapshot in time.[24]

Many see their spiritual life as a journey. The spiritual lives of most people are filled with twists, turns, and periods of confusion, as well as clarity. A single human experience rarely includes all the experiences and intensity (or lack of intensity) that phase and stage theories suggest. One life differs from another, and the impact of the same event differs from human to human. Hence, while metaphors such as journey, spiral, travel, and map may be helpful, every spiritual life is different and needs to explore its own metaphors to make sense of the questions and experiences.[25]

Some professional schools welcome a conversation on the topic of spirituality and health. Fortin and Barnett found that a growing number of medical schools offered courses on spirituality in medicine—seventeen schools offered such courses in 1994, and the number increased to eighty-four schools by 2004.[26] A course at the University of Michigan attempts to provide spiritual grounding to the notion of professionalism—spirituality in the sense of ultimate values such as love, beauty, hope, and truth.[27] The course encourages the practice of reflection to teach each student to "address the process of becoming a professional while

23. English et al., *Spirituality of Adult Education*, 97.

24. Tisdell, *Exploring Spirituality and Culture.*

25. English et al., *Spirituality of Adult Education and Training*, 123.

26. Fortin and Barnett, "Medical School Curricula."

27. Andre, "Moral Growth, Spirituality, and Activism," 80–94.

remaining a whole person—one whose values blend with the ideals of excellent professional practice, and whose professional practice embodies and demonstrates one's fully developed human excellences."[28]

AUTHENTICITY

Another professional characteristic that may be connected to empathy is authenticity. In his book *Jesus and the Disinherited*, Howard Thurman describes deception as a technique used by the weak against the strong. In many situations where control is on one side, the advantaged group assumes that they will be fooled and the weaker group uses deception as a survival strategy. Because questions of morality are left outside this equation, the individual emerges with no sense of ethical grounding. Practicing deception leads one to become a deception. Thurman recommends instead that the disadvantaged practice an overwhelming sincerity that leaves the dominant group with "no defense, with the edge taken away from the sense of prerogative."[29] What role does deception or inauthenticity play in student choices to undergo professional education? To what extent are authenticity and sincerity valued in a professional career?

Authenticity has been described as an attribute of presence. Watson notes that the degree of transpersonal caring is increased by the degree of genuineness and sincerity of the practitioner. When the nurse is not genuine, the patient is repelled, and this inauthenticity contributes to a state of disharmony (or illness). Watson describes the transpersonal caring process as an art that allows nurses to "call upon the inner depth of their own humanness and personal creativity as they realize the conditions of a person's soul and their own."[30]

Freya Zaltz describes authenticity as an aspect of the therapeutic relationship in counseling practice. Authenticity requires honesty, the moral need to care and be cared for, a self that can interact with others, and a self that is dynamic and changing. Inauthenticity, by contrast, focuses on self-fulfillment, dishonesty, and manipulation. Caring requires a shared understanding, not an individualistic striving. Zaltz argues that authenticity is essential in the relationship between learner and educa-

---

28. Fortin and Barnett, "Medical School Curricula."
29. Thurman, *Jesus and the Disinherited*, 73.
30. Watson, *Nursing*, 71.

tor.[31] When students in the classroom or professionals in their workplace recognize the interconnectedness of being, they can better visualize themselves as part of a community. Reaching a place of interconnection and inter-being can require a phase of cognitive dissonance—a stage of discomfort for the learner who needs to surrender core beliefs to adopt new ideas.

Parker Palmer describes how authenticity works in a teaching and learning situation. He believes that teachers and learners must respond to each other on the basis of a truth within. He writes, "The truth we are seeking, the truth that seeks us, lies ultimately in the community of being where we not only know but are known."[32] Palmer describes a balance between humility (willingness to listen) and faith (willingness to speak our own truth). Similarly, he poses reverence (respect for truth) as opposed to idolatry (treating the local as if it were absolute). Finally, love and openness to grace make possible the tensions in the above categories. Grace in this sense may serve as an inclusive term that covers a continuum, from divine grace to a gift received from the universe or from within. Irrespective of the origin of grace in an immanent or transcendent location, grace can function as a term that suggests mystery and gift. Teaching offers a form of spiritual discipline that can leave one open to the fruits of spiritual practice described above. Palmer recommends practicing silence, finding solitude, and practicing prayer.

RECIPROCITY

Reciprocity requires a sense of humility based on the realization that professional expertise does not allow one to dominate others. Reciprocity allows for the exchange of information and the attempt to understand the other's experience "as if" it were one's own, realizing that such precise knowledge of the other is out of reach. Although information about the client's experience is exchanged for the professional knowledge in the consultation, one type of information is not essentially more worthy than the other. Clients remain the experts on their experience, and the professional brings a different expertise (but not the sole expertise) to the consultation.

31. Zaltz, "Authenticity in Education."

32. Palmer, To Know as We Are Known, 90.

The encounter can be more than two solitary selves meeting to exchange information. Ann Chinnery and Heesoon Bai challenge the view of contemporary moral theorists who argue that empathy is a primary precondition for moral performance. Instead, they argue that the prevailing conception of modern subjectivity, with its privileging of an autonomous self, is an obstacle to the expression of empathy. They posit a reframing of the self-other binary, away from modern individualism towards different types of subjectivity—in this case, Emmanuel Levinas's prioritization of the other and the Buddhist deconstruction of the egoic self. Chinnery and Bai demonstrate how Levinas makes the concept of the other constitutive of selfhood.[33]

Moral agency thus requires the self to step down and to assume the needs of the other. By rejecting the autonomous subjectivity that has shaped much of Western philosophy since Descartes, the possibility emerges of a worldview and a moral stance that honors the relationality inherent in human subjectivity. The moral failure that allows the homeless to reside on the streets and the failure that allows the inequities of North American and global life would not be tolerated in a system where the situation of the other is part of the self. Rather than having empathy function as a precondition for moral performance, empathy would result from the shift in subjectivity and moral agency that this relationship between self and other necessitates.[34]

Nursing theory names this potential as therapeutic reciprocity, which allows an exchange of feelings, thoughts, and experiences. There is mutuality in this encounter that allows both the practitioner and the client to experience positive growth through the collaboration in the practitioner-client relationship. According to Patricia Marck, therapeutic reciprocity is "a mutual, collaborative, probabilistic, instructive, and empowering exchange of feelings, thoughts, and behaviors between nurse and client for the purpose of enhancing the human outcomes of the relationship for all concerned."[35] In the doctor-patient relationship, reciprocity is also considered relevant to the outcomes. However, since reciprocity can also be affected by a physician's appearing to be caring or authoritative, one can speculate that reciprocity should be accompanied by authenticity.[36]

33. Chinnery and Bai, "Altering Conceptions of Subjectivity," 86–96.

34. Ibid.

35. Marck, "Therapeutic Reciprocity," 49–59.

36. Gochman, *Health Behavior*.

PEDAGOGIES OF IMAGINATION

Hans Alma distinguishes between affective empathy, cognitive empathy, and interpretive empathy. These types of empathy may exist without being communicated. However, when they are communicated, there can be expressed empathy (either verbal or nonverbal), received and responsive empathy (when the other accepts the expressed empathy), or interactional empathy (when the empathizer and the other interact). For Alma, the optimum type of empathic understanding combines interactive and interpretive empathy to form a variation called dialogical-hermeneutical empathic understanding.[37]

What are the mechanisms for transmitting such empathy? Philosopher of education Maxine Greene argues that imagination allows us to cross the distance between the self and the other to picture alternative realities. This movement away from unquestioned consciousness to a self-reflective grasp of the role of the past in our lives is the heart of education. Rather than repeating endlessly the patterns of the past, new awareness and new beginnings are put into motion.

The imagination is essential to opening up the possibility of something new. Hannah Arendt laments the instrumental quality of modern culture wherein all the processes of the earth are man-made. Arendt says there are two mental operations involved in judgment: imagination and reflection. For Arendt, therefore, the enormity and unprecedented nature of totalitarianism have not destroyed, strictly speaking, our ability to judge. Rather, they have destroyed our accepted standards of judgment and conventional categories of interpretation and assessment, whether moral or political. And in this situation the only recourse is to appeal to the *imagination*—a capacity that allows us to view things in their proper perspective and to judge them without the benefit of a given rule or universal. For Arendt, the imagination enables us to create the distance that is necessary for an impartial judgment, while at the same time allowing for the closeness that makes understanding possible. In this way it makes possible our reconciliation with reality, even considering the tragic realities of history.

In a study of nursing knowledge, Holmes and Gastaldo contrast arborescent thought (a tree model that represents most of Western and humanist thought) and rhizomatic thought (which is multidirectional,

---

37. Alma, "Self-Development as a Spiritual Process," 61.

open-ended, and tolerant of ambivalence and chaos). They propose that the rhizomatic perspective enables creativity to happen—creativity that tolerates "diversified modes of thinking, visions of the world, values and knowledge development tools."[38] An attitude of openness, exploration, and newness can provide a practitioner with a willingness to find new ways of doing things and to truly become a lifelong learner. This openness is affected by the larger issues of knowledge production in a profession.

Hope is generated in the possibilities of imagination and creativity, and these open up in dialogical space, in contrast to hopelessness that results in silence. When an individual is given the appropriate tools, he or she can deal critically with social and personal reality. Greene notes that once distinct voices have been heard, the importance of shared beliefs can be attended to. These voices can emerge out of dialogue and regard for others' freedom. Community cannot be formed out of rational formulation or edict but only through the process of speaking and creating. Greene proposes the engagement of critical self-reflexiveness that involves critical thought from within shared human stories. The act of interrogating a lived world is far different from acting as an expert critique from outside a world. Greene believes that imagination is what makes empathy possible.[39]

Philosopher John Dewey believed in the need for common experience, which he felt was being undermined by the industrial age. Similarly, Alma notes that art and imagination can be important in "confronting people with new perspectives that differ profoundly from habitual ways of understanding their world."[40] Artists help us to view the world from different perspectives. Religion also can help provide a frame of reference to see the world differently. Alma notes, "one of the big challenges we face in our globalizing world is the training of our empathic abilities and the development of art and religion as languages of personal resonance that stimulate our mutual understanding."[41]

Ruth Richards argues that everyday creativity offers "new ways of thinking, of experiencing the world, and experiencing ourselves."[42]

38. Holmes and Gastaldo, "Rhizomatic Thought," 258–67.

39. Greene, *Releasing the Imagination*, 3–39.

40. Alma, "Self-Development as a Spiritual Process," 62.

41. Ibid., 63.

42. Richards, ed., *Everyday Creativity*, 5.

Creativity consists of originality and meaningfulness. Maslow's self-actualizing theory supported creativity. Other psychologists are also open to experience and to the role of ambiguity. Creativity has a moral dimension—Richards, for example, describes the benefits of creativity to the individual and society.

Rollo May distinguishes between creativity as "superficial aestheticism" and the authentic form of "bringing something new into being." In the creative process there must be a specific quality of engagement that contains an intensity of awareness. Creativity cannot be examined "as a subjective phenomenon" that attempts to figure out what goes on inside a person, since the process ultimately interrelates the person and the world.[43]

Something new is created in the process of creation, and both persons in the interaction are confronted with new perspectives. According to Alma, imagination is an important part of this process. It first enables us to take the perspective of others and to understand their desires and aims. Then it nourishes empathic understanding with perspectives that are not immediately given in the experiential world of the other, but that are derived from the societal, cultural, and historical context of the interaction.[44] Such engagement presumably can energize both sides of the professional encounter, as imagination enables connection and generates engagement rather than disconnection.

EDUCATIONAL INTERVENTIONS TO ENHANCE EMPATHY

Technical expertise and cognitive understanding are valued in professional education. Professional education is shaped by learner-centered objectives that move inexorably towards predetermined outcomes—success is thus marked in relation to these outcomes.

If the goal of professional education is to develop empathic practitioners, what types of pedagogies will be important to that process, and how will those outcomes be measured?

Hojat describes a variety of factors that impede the development of empathy in the education and practice of health professions, including the lack of role models and lack of "dedicated educational programs for

---

43. May, *Courage to Create*, 46.

44. Alma, "Self-Development as a Spiritual Process," 59–63.

nourishment of humanistic qualities in patient encounters."[45] In addition, changes in the health-care delivery system increase pressures for profit over relationship. Fear of malpractice impedes the formation of an empathic relationship between client and practitioner. Research on the effects of educational interventions on empathy remains inconclusive due to the difficulties associated with defining the parameters of empathy and the variety of scales used to measure empathy.

Empathy can be positively or negatively developed or demonstrate no change at all during the course of professional education. Hojat notes that the "extent to which the potential for empathy can be actualized or enhanced in a particular person will depend on the interaction of several factors, including the person's constitutional makeup, early life experiences, motivation, and a facilitating environment, as well as exposure to specific educational programs."[46] Such a complex interaction of factors enhancing empathic engagement requires a strong commitment by professional faculties and schools.

What kinds of activities and pedagogical methods can help develop empathy? Methods include parental training, workshops, perspective-taking exercises, role-playing, communication skills, films and videos, and role modeling. Hojat notes that when medical students and nurses work and communicate together, the collaborative professional relationship improves significantly. Increased understanding of patients and coworkers in this case leads to increased collaboration in the workplace. Surveying a number of empathy-training programs for health-care professionals reveals that organizations generally attempt to improve interpersonal skills in order to enhance the capacity for empathy. Many of the programs to enhance empathy focus on encouraging the students to place themselves in the client's situation, using cognitive skills (the clinical aspects of a disease) and emotional skills (imagining the patient's experience with a disease). Interprofessional dialogue and training may be essential to enhance empathy.

Communication studies and small group work have demonstrated that interventions can improve doctor's abilities to communicate with patients and to exhibit deeper levels of empathy.[47] Engaging the imagi-

45. Hojat, *Empathy in Patient Care*, 180.

46. Ibid., 80–82.

47. Suchman, "What Makes the Patient-Doctor Relationship Therapeutic?" 125–30; Balint and Shelton, *Regaining the Initiative*, 887–91.

nation is key to being able to understand the "as if" situation. In addition, intercultural skills help professionals cross the boundaries of the known to the unknown. Intercultural sensitivity and communication demand a deep awareness of one's emotional reactions.

PEDAGOGIES OF TRANSFORMATION TO ENHANCE EMPATHY

There are a variety of challenges to add empathy-related skills, knowledge, and attitudes into the curriculum. Although outcomes-based curricula are increasingly becoming standard in a variety of educational settings, certain learning moments, such as providing empathic patient care, do not easily lend themselves to evaluation and to productivity analyses. H. Edward Everding and Lucinda Huffaker propose "that educating adults for empathy involves the transformation of cognitive perspectives through expanding, deepening, broadening, and enriching persons' understandings of themselves, one another's, and the traditions and shaping visions of the faith communities of which they are a part."[48] Their research examines development and identity formation, and they observe that the distinguishing feature of relationships that nurture selfhood and clarify identity is their "mutuality of empathy (compare to unreciprocated empathy which is domination)."[49] The educational implications of their approach include role-playing (imagining being the other); listening, as in compassionate listening; journaling; and engaging in encounters and immersion experiences.

How does transformative education claim to effect change? It changes the frames of reference of the adult learner by focusing on the interrelationship between personal change and learning. Jack Mezirow teaches that critical reflection is part of the process of changing habits of mind. In the process of professional training, students encounter their frames of reference through dialogue, critical reflection, and action; they develop increased competence in reading context, understanding diversity, reflecting on personal responses, taking action, and reflecting critically on the effectiveness of that action. The process provides the students with skills that can potentially form part of a lifelong practice and contribute to improved self-understanding, enhanced efficacy, increased

48. Everding and Huffaker, "Educating Adults," 419.
49. Ibid., 422.

openness to learning, increased collaborative learning, and improved ability to adapt to complex and changing systems.[50]

Curry-Stevens studied the use of transformative education to advance social justice issues among privileged groups. She studied twenty community-based practitioners who worked in the field of transformative education. One quarter of the learners commented that the process of working through pedagogy for the privileged entailed a spiritual conversion from an individual orientation to an interdependent connection concerned for humanity. Pedagogy for the privileged also activates the following emotions: grief, fear, guilt, discomfort, as well as excitement, anticipation, and joy.[51] When the educational process induces guilt, there can be a point where the learner can feel a debilitating amount of responsibility for privilege and for the inequality it represents. This can result in intense emotions that can prevent the learner from acting. An awareness of empathic processing attempts to move students beyond liberal guilt with its affective overload. Action that might proceed from such overload may colonize or sympathize with little critical self-reflection. Brené Brown has studied the workings of guilt and shame, particularly among women, and observes that shame obstructs connectedness and diminishes our ability to be empathic. Shame triggers a response that moves from shame to anger to blame, and the entire cycle inhibits connectedness.[52]

Changing awareness is the first step in teaching about privilege—the next step is building a commitment to engage in social justice practices. The necessary cognitive shift that makes this possible includes unlearning and relearning. Students should be cautioned to expect a degree of cognitive dissonance as their belief systems and self-image may be radically altered in this process.

Curry-Stevens presents a transformation model for privileged learners that changes Freire's focus on the oppressed in which the movement is from individual experience to awareness of structural and systemic issues.[53] Her model also allows for all learners to be validated for their own experience of suffering before they can recognize themselves as privileged. At this stage, learners may build empathy for themselves

50. Mezirow, *Learning as Transformation.*
51. Curry-Stevens, "New Forms of Transformative Education."
52. Brown, *I Thought It Was Just Me.*
53. Freire, *Pedagogy of the Oppressed.*

and for each other in their suffering in order to create common ground. Only after prior stages have been achieved can one ask the learner to understand him- or herself as implicated in the oppression of others. The next four steps of her model involve building agency to undertake action, since awareness alone does not lead to action.[54]

REFLECTION AS PART OF THE PROCESS OF EMPATHIC DEVELOPMENT

Many professional training programs use reflection as a process to develop skills that can be useful in empathic development. Three phases of the reflective process include awareness of uncomfortable thoughts or feelings, critical analysis of personal feelings and reflective knowledge, and perspective transformation.[55] The process follows Mezirow's concept of emancipatory learning—an organized effort to help the learner challenge presuppositions, explore alternative perspectives, transform ways of understanding, and act on new perspectives.[56]

Reflection may help students recognize that they are part of an interconnected universe—a capacity Miller describes as compassionate knowing. Students are also encouraged to encounter and reflect on suffering.[57] Courses examining suffering for nurses include a fourteen-week interdisciplinary course.[58] The course attempts to help students improve their ability to recognize the suffering of others and respond to it in such a way as to optimally relieve or alleviate a patient's distress.

Suffering can thus be its own teacher, both in encountering one's own suffering or the suffering of the other. However, this encounter must be accompanied by a process of critical reflection. In a study of the role of emotion in socially just teaching, Sharon Chubbuck and Michalinos Zembylas note that teachers and teachers in training need to engage and reflect on emotion. They observe, "By learning how to develop practices of critical emotional praxis in their teaching, pre-service and in-service teachers can begin to create spaces for interrogating unjust and exclu-

---

54. Curry-Stevens, "New Forms of Transformative Education," 53.

55. Atkins and Murphy, "Reflection," 1188–92.

56. Mezirow, *Transformative Dimensions*.

57. Miller, "Learning from a Spiritual Perspective," 95–102.

58. Kazanowski et al., "Silence of Suffering," 195–203.

sionary teaching."[59] Teacher educators need to address the significance of emotion in sustaining or dismantling structures of power, privilege, racism, and colonization. Those structures depend on withholding certain emotional responses (such as grief, remorse, compassion, and caring) toward certain groups of people deemed other. To confront the pain and exclusion felt by many, teachers and students need to engage in what Boler called a pedagogy of discomfort or a pedagogy of suffering.[60]

The process of reflection and writing has been increasingly used as a tool to encourage practitioners to be fully present in the clinical situation and to monitor their reactions for their learning. Charon argues that health professionals should be equipped with the skills that allow them to understand the patient's narrative. Then, through their own powers of reflection and clinical imagination, they can appreciate the situation of the patient. In the end, she notes, "They can then, with deep empathy, name the suffering they see, offer themselves humbly as one who recognizes, who listens, and who cares."[61]

JOURNALING AND PORTFOLIO DEVELOPMENT

Reflecting on learning can involve the use of journaling or portfolios. Portfolios allow both the instructor and the student to track change through documenting the student's learning and insights. One can differentiate between the phenomenological method (how one orients to life experience) and the hermeneutic (how one interprets life's texts).[62] Van Maanen proposes that hermeneutic phenomenological research can investigate experience as we live it.[63] Some of the literature distinguishes between reflection as occurring from within the process and reflection that happens after the process is finished. Adaptive leadership requires an ability to reflect-in-action as well as reflect after the fact.

How can this approach be adapted to outcomes-based evaluation methods? Evaluating such learning requires a complex set of skills on the part of the instructor as well. In each course or discipline, the objectives for the course must match the reflective assignments so that the

---

59. Chubbuck and Zembylas, "Emotional Ambivalence," 284.
60. Boler and Zembylas, "Discomforting Truths."
61. Charon, *Stories Matter*, 103.
62. Maich, "'Becoming' through Reflection," 309–24.
63. Van Maanen, *Researching Lived Experience*.

purposes match the instructor's intent and follow transparent and measurable standards of evaluation. Mentoring reflective processes is not the same as teaching content—in the former, the teacher must be willing to engage in the same vulnerability and personal growth that he or she demands of the student. Both must be able to tolerate the ambiguity of the learner-learner experience. For students who demand certainty and prefer imposed learning, this can be an uncomfortable moment. For teachers who enjoy their authority and power, this may require a radical shift in method.

In describing pedagogies that inform clergy education, Charles Foster claims that pedagogies of contextual encounter develop in students an appreciation of the other on the other's terms. Foster notes, "This capacity for contextual self-knowledge, however, is the corollary of 'getting to know the other in their otherness,' which similarly requires learning how to allow others 'to define themselves' and how to approach them in their diversity with 'respect and reverence.'"[64]

Critical thinking results in an awareness of the "diversity of values, behaviors, social structures and artistic forms in the world."[65] Developing critical thinking depends on becoming aware of the assumptions that shape our interpretations of the world. Sometimes critical reflection can arise out of a negative trigger or crisis, but in other cases joy can be a trigger. Critical thinking is central to the work of adult education. Critical reflection attempts to create conditions under which people can learn to love one another and urges us "to create the conditions under which each person is respected, valued, and heard."[66] Some of the methods of teaching critical thinking skills include critical questioning, critical incident exercises, criteria analysis, critical debate, and crisis-decision simulations. How can we help people to imagine alternatives? Some of the methods include brainstorming, envisioning alternative futures, developing preferred scenarios, futures invention, goal formulation, indicator invention, scenario construction, and aesthetic triggers.

---

64. Foster et al., eds., *Educating Clergy*, 144.

65. Brookfield, *Developing Critical Thinkers*, 5.

66. Brookfield, *Becoming a Critically Reflective Teacher*, 26.

BORDER PEDAGOGY

Henry Giroux describes teaching as a process that requires both thinking and practice—dual skills that might relate to the cognitive and affective components of empathic engagement.[67] His view matches Donald Schön's work on the reflective practitioner.[68] Doyle and Singh argue that teachers can collaborate with their students to transform lived experience—a transformation that happens in institutions and relationships in small ways over time.[69] Giroux's concept of border pedagogy describes the border as the epistemological, political, cultural, and social margins that structure the language of history, power, and difference. Educators have to learn to cross borders so they can understand otherness on its own terms. Teaching thus creates a space where students learn to attend to and be responsible for the narratives of others. According to Goleman, paying attention allows us to build an emotional connection; without attention, empathy would not have a chance.[70]

Professionals face the risk that unchecked empathy and affective overload can put them at risk for burnout or stress. Working with specific populations, such as traumatized individuals, can provide severe challenges for practitioners. In such cases, empathy must be carefully monitored. Judith Herman underlines the need for support for the therapist when she writes, "Unless the therapist has adequate support to bear this grief, she will not be able to fulfill her promise to bear witness and will withdraw emotionally from the therapeutic alliance."[71] However, many practitioners deal with complex family situations and are exposed to many types of suffering. To witness and interact with this suffering over time requires not only empathic connection but also deep spiritual care to prevent burnout or detachment.

Barry Kanpol and Peter McLaren question how one can develop empathy that "allows for a unification of minds, a form of intersubjectivity, despite the multiple and clearly confusing differences between these particular peoples."[72] This proposed pedagogy includes an empathic

---

67. Giroux, "War against Children," 3.

68. Schön, *Reflective Practitioner*.

69. Doyle and Singh, *Reading and Teaching Henry Giroux*.

70. Goleman, *Social Intelligence*, 51.

71. Herman, *Trauma and Recovery*, 144.

72. Kanpol and McLaren, "Multiculturalism and Empathy," 179.

incorporation of the diverse other that establishes similarities without losing multiple differences. This border pedagogy unifies the centers and margins of power. Empathy is an essential part of this pedagogy, where educators recover their own memories and experiences and reconstruct them in a framework of mutuality and care, while celebrating the individual differences that each brings to the interaction.

In the next chapter, we will examine the formation of compassionate communities. These communities include the professional culture of learning organizations, professional practice settings, and the communities in which individual clients find their home.

QUESTIONS FOR FURTHER DISCUSSION

1. Find an organization that works for justice. Research its mission and values. How does it accomplish its mission?

2. Compare charity to justice. What are the differences? As a professional, what would be the difference in your relationships working out of a charity versus a justice model?

3. Describe the diversity of clients in your workplace. What do you know about the cultures that you serve? Choose one of these cultural groups and find out what you can about their presence in the neighborhood.

4. Are there diverse faith communities in your neighborhood? Can you locate them? Visit a place of worship and find out something about the members there.

5. Interview someone about his or her faith experience. How do they describe it? Compare their description to that of a faith-development theorist such as James Fowler or Sharon Daloz Parks.

6. How have your beliefs changed over time? Draw a life map, dividing your life into stages and marking significant events and the progression of your beliefs.

7. What place do imagination and creativity have in your practice? Define creativity and how it impacts your professional life.

8. Have you had educational experiences that were transformative? Describe one and how it transformed you.

9. Many of us have privileges that we are often unaware of. Draw a map of the various networks and groups that you belong to, including school, athletics, and other activities.

10. Recall an experience you had with difference. Describe the encounter and how you felt. Did this experience create a barrier to your understanding of the client, or were you motivated to learn more about the client?

6

Empathic Communities

Healing refers to the restoration and rehabilitation of persons to their full power and vitality in the life of the community. Sickness, then does not refer primarily to physical pain as much as to the inability to be fully, honorably and seriously engaged in the community in all its decisions and celebrations."[1]

WALTER BRUEGGEMAN DESCRIBES HEALTH as the restoration of people to community. Such a definition resonates with the Hebrew Bible's use of the word *shalom* to describe wholeness. Much of the work of professions involves this restoration to wholeness, whether through education, health, or pastoral or spiritual interventions. These interventions may involve seeking solutions for the physical place of people in community (for example, the homeless or insufficiently housed); the need for work, food, and recreation (retraining, community gardens, or sport); the spiritual care of diverse populations (chaplaincy, advocacy, or solace); health care (prevention, access, health promotion, and nutrition), and education (literacy, creativity, and access to advanced training).

In this chapter we will look at the definition of community and then attempt to address how professional education can prepare students to restore individuals to community or build a community's capacity through empathy. In addition, the experience of professional training can itself be a model for the experience of community. Thus, we will examine how students might experience community during their professional training.

---

1. Brueggeman, *Peace*, 199.

WHAT IS COMMUNITY?

Community is derived from the Latin *communitas* (with/together) and *mundus* (gift). The term community is sometimes used to refer to an ideal that has not yet been realized ("We need to build community") or to refer to a shared group, fellowship, town, or organization. "Community" can describe a group of people who share housing, a profession, a sport, or a job. Although physical shared space is often assumed in the definition, virtual communities and social networks increasingly define the boundaries of community both online and across physical space.

The existence of community suggests that individual interests have been transcended in favor of a greater purpose or meaning that is inclusive of difference but embraces a shared mission. In the previous chapter, we saw how border pedagogy included both the centers and the margins and incorporated diversities while seeking a common understanding or purpose.

When tasks are completed and goals are achieved, the community sets new goals—a community thus is defined by change as much as it upholds tradition. Integral to community is the ability to communicate and to achieve shared understanding despite cultural or language differences or physical barriers to communication. The community builds and enacts shared memory and celebrates this through stories and rituals.[2] Ultimately the community has the capacity to rejoice and to mourn together. The sharing of grief can create new communities. The building of a peace garden to commemorate the deaths of young people after a violent Toronto summer in 1999 brought together strangers with a common purpose. For some, community represents a feeling of being at home and being accepted, whereas for others, community represents a point in the past from which they hope to escape. Although the purposes of community are dynamic, community can be experienced as static for those who yearn for transformation or to be perceived in different ways than the community perceives them. Others are displaced by violence and war and risk everything to find a place where they can begin again.

Peter Block notes that the challenge to community is to transform isolation and self-interest into hospitable community. Two questions that might structure that conversation include: what do we want to create together that would make a difference? and what can we create together

---

2. See, for example, Anderson and Foley, *Mighty Stories, Dangerous Rituals.*

than we cannot create alone?[3] Block distinguishes between human and political suffering. Human suffering is the inevitable pain that is part of human life, including illness and death. The other kind of pain is political suffering and is avoidable, including poverty, homelessness, violence, and neighborhoods in distress. This suffering occurs as a result of our disconnectedness and the imbalance of power and resources. He notes that "when we are unrelated to those whose lives are so different from ours, suffering increases."[4] Professionals may encounter both types of suffering and may also experience the disconnectedness that separates them from the inhabitants of a community that they are attempting to serve. Hospitals that serve disadvantaged neighborhoods, churches that become the physical home for the homeless, and schools that struggle with complex problems and little support suffer from empathic fatigue as the resources never match the demand.

The term "community" is often invoked with a certain amount of romantic longing; in reality, isolation and hatred may characterize some communities. Even shared suffering may increase isolation and distrust. Shared culture, tradition, history are no guarantee that a willingness to build community will emerge. According to Thurman, the misunderstanding that fosters hatred often begins where there is contact without fellowship. Thurman warns against sentimentality that masquerades as fellowship. Such sentimentality can structure the relations of faith communities, learning communities, and housing communities and distort relationships when the dominant group defines reality for the less powerful. One's identity as an individual or part of a group can never be fully realized in such an inequitable arrangement.

Distinguishing between solidarity with the poor versus merely feeling sorry for them, bell hooks observes that privileged people often seek to help the poor without changing their hatred of or contempt for them.[5] The shift in critical consciousness that Paulo Freire describes as necessary requires a shift in the privileged classes as well, lest patterns of domination continue to be reproduced. Both the non-poor and the poor require transformation to produce alternate ways of thinking, feeling, and acting. As Thurman reminds us, those who have been dominated have an embodied fear that must be unlearned at the physiological as

3. Block, *Community*, 127.

4. Ibid., 164.

5. hooks, *Where We Stand*.

well as the cognitive level.[6] Building community with partners of diverse backgrounds demands a willingness to be vulnerable, to share experiences, and to shape a common purpose. Creativity in community building is an essential feature in order to tolerate ambiguity, chaos, and loss of control as something new and unpredictable emerges.

LOSS OF A COMMON WORLD

Community depends on a commonality of purpose, a commonality that can occasionally be lost. Writers, philosophers, artists, and others have described the loss of our common world through technology, migration, war, natural disasters, domination, and other causes. A shift in circumstances can force families to leave their homes, their countries, and their family members. Economic, political, religious, and personal factors contribute to the loss of a common home. When trauma accompanies this loss, a variety of physical manifestations and emotional aftereffects can interrupt individual functioning, which in turn can be experienced and inherited by successive generations. In the illness experience, a patient can experience chaos that has no beginning or ending.

Illness can rob a person of a common world. C. M. Hertogh described the loss of a common world in the lives of patients with dementia in a nursing home. Such a loss creates challenges for professionals who seek to care for these patients. He observed three features of the loss of a common world of shared meaning: the dilemma(s) of truth speaking and truthfulness; the struggle to hold on to reciprocity in care giving; and the paradoxes of normality nurses face in their treatment of people with dementia. In order to help caregivers cope with these problems, the study recommended that supportive work be done with nurses.[7]

War, political violence, terrorism, and other forms of dominance can result in social suffering and the destruction of communities. This violence can be sudden and intense or slow and prolonged. Veena Das examines the way in which individuals and communities attempt to recreate normality and address the future in the face of social suffering. When communities experience suffering, how do individuals within them, as well as the communities as a whole, move forward to re-imagine their well-being? Thurman suggests that not deception, nor fear,

6. Thurman, *Jesus and the Disinherited*.

7. Hertogh, "Loss of a Common Shared World," 265–72.

nor hatred help a community to face its oppressors. A community must re-imagine its future, while retaining traditions and moving towards making a public sphere wherein notions of citizenship can be renegotiated. When communities have suffered, healing "means repair but it also means transformation—transformation to a different moral state."[8] Loss of relational abilities and disappearance of an ability to imagine a future are characteristics of traumatized individuals as well as communities.[9]

CREATING A COMMON WORLD

Maxine Greene suggests that the solution to caring for the world and the people in it derives not from therapeutic education or expert advice, but from communities generating ideas collectively that will lead to social repair. The ethical basis of community building and of education relies on bringing people together into "norm-governed situations" in which they discover a sense of obligation or responsibility. Such caring and capacity building can derive either from their innate sense of caring or from their own conceptions of justice and equity. The starting point, whether from empathy or from principle, does not matter to Greene. But the end result would be cooperative action to help heal society. Education, she argues, should bring students into situations where they discover this sense of obligation and caring for community and should address their role as citizens.[10]

But where in education or in society in general can this kind of collaboration and discussion happen? Merely describing or observing does not fit the process that Greene is recommending—in fact, it is a knowing that leads to doing. As described earlier in chapters 3 and 4, regarding suffering is only one part of knowing. The second part involves appropriate and empathic response to suffering. Instead of allowing students to be overwhelmed by the global problems of the world (and consequently doing nothing as a result), Greene recommends a focus on the local and everyday. She believes that individuals, in the course of conversation, will transcend their individual perspectives in favor of a shared, norm-governed world. Because a common Truth cannot bind believers in a pluralistic society to guide these encounters, Greene be-

8. Das et al., eds., *Remaking a World,* 23.

9. Jones, *Trauma and Grace.*

10. Greene, *Releasing the Imagination,* 65–66.

lieves that an ethical basis will provide the common ground. Without a transcendent value of Truth or the Good, she suggests that the focus on what is shared in a lived life will open up the possibility of a plurality that can be enlarged so that "more people will become willing to choose as the absolute the right of human beings to act in their freedom."[11]

NARRATIVE, RITUAL, AND MEMORY

Storytelling is one of the ways that we move from lived experience to meaning making and ultimately to the shared experience that shapes community. Reading literature can release the imagination in a way that allows one to revisit the past and interact with the present. The reshaping of the past into the future releases one from the habitual and allows for new understandings. According to Lewis and Sandra Hinchman, stories help create a community. Narratives, they argue, "explain a group to itself, legitimate its deeds and aspirations, and provide important benchmarks for non-members trying to understand the group's cultural identity."[12]

The work of imagining and reading works of literature open the vision of the reader to things that "might be." Students need to engage imagination and metaphor in order to have the tools to make sense out of the things they learn and to be able to question the habitual. The lack of monolithic narrative or grand truth suggests that in a postmodern sense, all are homeless and must create a home out of the practices of speaking and acting to create what it is that is the common world. Story engages both the listener and the teller in acts of mutuality as they listen and imagine the world through the experience of the other. Listening validates the experience "as if" it were one's own. Story and ritual offer the potential for empathic connection.

NAMING AND COUNTERING UPROOTEDNESS

Philosopher Hannah Arendt (1906-1975) described worldlessness as the disappearance of individuality. Humanity, she observed, has become homeless in the modern world. Narrative is how we create the common world, and to be without the past or memory is to lose one's sense of self-identity.

---

11. Ibid., 70.

12. Hinchman and Hinchman, eds., *Memory, Identity, Community*, 235.

Arendt valued an impartiality she attributed to the Greeks, who learned that the world we have in common could be seen from a diverse number of standpoints. Modern and scientific objectivity, she observed, does not have this capacity of entertaining different points of view. Political action derives from individuals acting together on a common project, but when such projects are remembered, they are remembered as the deeds of great individuals.

Arendt described the essence of education as natality—the fact that humans are born into the world and the world is constantly renewed through birth. The purpose of education is to prepare children for the task of renewing a common world. Natality offers the opportunity to innovate through action and provides the rationale for education.[13] Natasha Levinson reminds us that although natality suggests that the world can be renewed, the capacity for action must be nurtured. The world that education supports is produced by humans and conditions them with a resulting plurality. The principle of natality preserves hopefulness since each new individual brings the capacity for innovation and potential change. Education is important because teachers can protect individual creativity while preserving the public world—education can create the conditions for the setting right of the world.[14]

Human action was described by Arendt as unpredictable, in contrast to technology and bureaucratic processes that value control and efficiency. For education, this means honoring individual action on behalf of the common world that can transcend local and individual interests and interest groups.

Politics that involve acting and speaking require the presence of others and a common space where many gather.[15] The faculty of judgment is not a private estimation but an "enlarged way of thinking that . . . knows how to transcend its individual limitations . . . and needs the presence of others 'in whose place' it must think, whose perspectives it must take into consideration, and without whom it never has the opportunity to operate at all. Judgment requires the presence of others and may be a political task in which the 'sharing-the-world-with-others' comes to pass."[16] Judgment can free the individual from narcissism and

13. Arendt, *Between Past and Future*, 196.
14. Levinson, "Paradox of Natality," 11–36.
15. Arendt, *Between Past and Future*.
16. Ibid., 221.

self-interest, but it is opposed to objectivity and impartial judgment, which maintain an individual and neutral stance. When participants come together in common space to participate in a shared purpose, all participants must agree on the principle of equality. Because of her experience of totalitarianism, Arendt was concerned that individuals would feel free to speak in the face of new evil that might arise.

Simone Weil also perceived troubling tendencies in the modern world that resulted in uprootedness and alienation. Uprootedness results from military conquest, economic domination, and money. In her book *The Need for Roots* Weil describes order as one of the soul's needs. Individuals in the modern world facing incompatible obligations could only respond by desiring the good that was common to all humans at all times. As humans, we owe respect to community because it provides food for human souls. Weil delivered strong criticism against the educational system in France because she believed that technical science and specialization had replaced the knowledge of classical traditions. Weil believed that the spirituality of work should be a core value of civilization. When an individual empties her soul, she allows eternal Wisdom to enter into it. Work allows for a form of obedience that allows grace to enter. Both death and labor are part of the realm of necessity, which one can either revolt against or accept.[17]

CO-CREATORS OF A COMMON WORLD

Action and contemplation are part of the creation of a common world. For Parker Palmer this world contains a hidden wholeness. One of the negative effects of education, according to Palmer, is that people lack the capacity to help create community and thus become manipulators rather than co-creators of this common world. We need to examine the inner self which gives rise to the drive for dominance. To learn is to face transformation and to enter into relationship.

One of the disadvantages of the specialized training of professionals, Parker observes, is that the isolation ensured by this specialized knowledge allows them to judge their work by exclusive professional standards. Professionals or knowledge specialists are consequently isolated in their specialty and do not think about the pattern that they have to fit their work into. Work that is professionalized is no longer subject to

---

17. Weil, *Need for Roots*, 286.

the standards of community life, religion, health, or any other standards that can cause us to ask the right questions about what we are doing. If you are an isolated specialist, you might never ask what a proposed innovation will do to your community because you are not aware of having a community. Specialists are sometimes very selfless people, working long hours with altruistic motives, but Palmer warns that if one works too long in isolation, one loses the sense of limits or the sense of the effect of one's work on other people.

Palmer has written about professional training in terms of community, which he defines as the capacity for relatedness—not only to the world, but also to things of the spirit. In addition to the ability to think critically or to tolerate ambiguity, professionals need the capacity for relatedness. Community in this sense allows for conflict and for honest discussion because it is held together by love. Such a notion of love is very different from a sentimentalized notion of love and community. Palmer notes that community is the place where the person you least want to live with always lives. Those who dwell in dense urban spaces understand the challenges that these relationships can bring.[18]

In the classroom, the ethos of competitive individualism robs students of the ability to form meaningful community. Learning culture in higher education teaches one to become a manipulator of the other rather than a co-creator. Despite its rhetoric of valuing collaboration, professional education generally rewards competition. Palmer suggests that reflective work requires one to confront and embrace one's inner demons as sources of strength. Neither a strong nor a weak ego can contribute to the relational interaction with the world, as he observes in the following: "Both destroy our capacity for right action because both proceed from the same mistaken premise: the assumption that effective action requires us to be relevant, powerful, and spectacular, that only by being can we have a real impact on the world."[19]

The creation of community embodies design elements that facilitate interaction and cooperation. Thackara suggests that we need to rethink spaces, places and communities "in order to better exploit the dynamic potential of networked collaboration."[20] He concludes that creating community is about "copresence through time of bodies and the emer-

---

18. Palmer, *To Know as We Are Known*, 114.

19. Palmer, *Active Life*, 114.

20. Thackara, *In the Bubble*, 99.

gence of shared meaning as we interact with each other in meaningful activities."[21] During the hospitalization of his young daughter, Thackara realized that medical knowledge for doctors and nurses is embodied, which means that workplaces should take this kind of knowledge into account.

Design elements allow for interaction and cooperation that facilitate hospitality to the community. Relationality is inherent in human interaction whether in illness or health. Sociologist Arthur Frank, for example, describes the ethical choice assumed in the relational understandings of the body and illness. Frank suggests that the monadic model of medicine fits well with medicine's emphasis on individual achievement, whereas the dyadic body represents an ethical choice.[22] Stories become an essential part of establishing the relational and ethical nature of the illness experience, both for the teller and the listener. Memory is a responsibility to be guarded because "as it is told, it becomes witness and reaches beyond the individual into the consciousness of the community."[23]

EMPATHY AND INTERCONNECTEDNESS IN HIGHER EDUCATION

College experience in the past offered students varying degrees of community. In contemporary higher education, the diverse values and beliefs of a pluralistic culture have to be negotiated creatively. As Jon Dalton notes, "We are not advocating a restoration of traditional religiosity but a conception of community that embraces the diversity of religious and spiritual beliefs, as well as their shared values and moral ideas."[24] The decline of community in some colleges and universities is a result of the division of campus life by specialization, individualism, and entrepreneurialism. Commuting students or those working full- or part-time jobs have little opportunity to participate in community building. Whether in undergraduate or professional education, recognition of spiritual needs as the longing for mutuality and connection might contribute to an experience of wholeness or connectedness that ties individual hopes and

21. Ibid., 109.

22. Frank, *Wounded Storyteller*.

23. Ibid., 63–64.

24. Dalton, "Integrating Spirit and Community," 165–86.

learning to a sense of connection to the university and the community as a whole.

Further research would be required to ascertain the extent to which students experience disconnection in professional education. Do schools focus on transmitting information and ignore or avoid discussion of the deeper spiritual issues that affect students' lives and performance as professionals? Connectedness and empathy in professional training and practice relies both on mentoring and organizational design that allows individuals to form community.

One might argue that schooling based on competition destroys connectedness. In professional education, competition begins prior to admission and continues. Even when grades are not assigned, students compete for scarce resources, such as placements in choice practica, attention of tutors, and references from well-known professors. Education rarely offers alternatives to competitive interaction—academic performance is generally rewarded over collaborative behavior or service initiatives. In fields where service is valued, students lead a divided life when they compete for academic achievement and attempt to meet the service ideals in their spare time. Such a division places the responsibility on students to find a balance that does not in fact exist among the faculty or in the curriculum or learning culture of the school itself. In addition, habits of reflection and possibilities for integration are eliminated by the frantic pace of the day.

FORMS AND MEANINGS OF COMMUNITY
IN HIGHER EDUCATION

Robert Nash describes three levels of educational community as moral worlds. First is the personal, in which connections with family, friends, and one's interior life form the core of belonging. Second, he describes the experiences of campus life and relationships such as those with peers, faculty, and administrators. The third form of community is the broader societal realm where citizenship, patriotism, and individual rights and responsibilities define the roles and values of a communal life.[25] Dalton describes a fourth level as the global dimension of community life.[26] Such distinctions are part of the assumed culture of higher education;

25. Nash, *Spirituality, Ethics and Teaching.*
26. Dalton, "Integrating Spirit and Community," 174.

however, students might benefit from reflection on those moral communities and their place in them. Overlapping and contradictory commitments can undermine one's ability to form connection or to engage in empathic relationship. Such conflicts will presumably continue into a professional career.

Sharon Daloz Parks describes how young adults find meaning in their lives and in a shared future. Part of this meaning-making requires students to be mentored to become citizen-leaders in the new commons. The community that mentors young people offers hospitality to their emerging selves.[27] Higher education can provide this type of mentoring community to the formation of critical adult faith. Mentoring for professional education demands attention not only to the ethical questions of professional life but also to the potential contribution of each profession to the strength of our common life.[28] The experience of community in education leads to the dreams of community and of the importance of the commons for young adults and professionals who will take the lead in caring for the world.

John Dewey wrote in reaction to both regimented schooling and expanding industrialism when he envisioned individuals engaged in collaboration to solve shared problems.[29] Community comes into being through communicating and sharing experience. As Walter Fisher explains, Dewey believed that community was not a mode of nation-state governance but a "mode of associated living, of conjoint communicated experience."[30]

What would a caring community in a higher-education or professional-training classroom look like? Professional schools tend to reward achievement more than relational abilities. Awards and prizes for both students and teachers are generally given on the basis of academic merit. Collaborative work assignments are often resisted by students—not only do they fear a lower grade when partnered with someone who does not show the same ability, but they prefer to work on their own. Small-group process is often resisted since students prefer content to be given by lecture as a more convenient mode of learning. In order to shift to a collaborative model, classroom spaces and grade allocation would need

27. Daloz Parks, *Big Questions, Worthy Dreams*, 93.
28. Ibid., 175.
29. Schutz, "Contesting Utopianism," 93–125.
30. Fisher, "Narration, Reason, and Community," 311.

to be reconsidered. Many professional schools have done so with the implementation of case study or problem-based learning activities—but others find it difficult to change the individualist models of learning that have been in place for decades.

Shelley Kessler describes teaching presence as being fully present, having an open heart, and maintaining discipline.[31] Do those school-based values have any relevance to teaching in higher education or in a professional school climate? Even when an academic community values connectedness, it is possible that the hidden curriculum cancels it out in favor of isolation and competition. Privileging certain behaviors and knowledge over others is a subtle way for professional-education programs to instill messages about individualism and competition; such messages are not easily overcome. Schools that express openness to diversities may still adhere to a learning culture that is based in Western and white ways of knowing. Willingness to critically examine the implicit curriculum of a professional school or program demands scrutiny of the assumptions of the learning community—an examination that is far more complex than merely a review of the curriculum. Indeed, the learning culture as a whole, including the curriculum content, the pedagogy, and the organizational ethos, can include or exclude students either intentionally or unintentionally.

Alfie Kohn observes that a true community is not a collective. He refers to philosopher Martin Buber, who writes that a community "not only preserves and nourishes the individuals who compose it but also underscores the relationships among these individuals."[32] Attempts to create community or to force community-building exercises on a group can fall flat.

Community can also be encouraged outside of the classroom in the activities of the school and in the contact a school maintains with its students over time. The application of learning to practice and the challenge to keep up with ever-changing bodies of knowledge can provide opportunities for continuing levels of community for professional-school graduates. Even in continuing education, community can be sustained by recognition of and commitment to a common purpose.

Buber describes community as the realm of the "between" where the I and Thou meet. He emphasizes that community must be built on

31. Kessler, "Teaching Presence."

32. Kohn, *Beyond Discipline*, 108.

authentic interaction with people whose intention is to establish a living relationship. The actualization of community in Buber's thinking relies on the human capacity to enter the "in-between" and to be in relation to others through dialogic communication.[33]

Based on his presumption that humans are basically storytellers, Fisher proposes narration as a conceptual frame for community. The stories we tell each other are symbolic actions—words and deeds—that have sequence and meaning for those who live, create, or interpret them. Living within these stories provides the common life of a community. He writes, "Regardless of form, discursive or non-discursive texts are meant to give order to life by inducing others to dwell in them to establish ways of living in common, in intellectual and spiritual communities in which there is confirmation for the story that constitutes one's life."[34]

If stories are essential to the process of community building, where in professional education are stories exchanged and experienced? Increasingly, contemplation and reflection are added to individual courses to allow students to process new information and to account for change in their own perspectives. Sharing stories, however, requires a common space that affirms individual perspective and suggests that difference can foster a commonality when hospitality is the norm. Why are these skills important for professional students?

Teachers, nurses, clergy, and doctors may interact with individuals as well as their communities. Schools, churches, and community health centers are sites where the work of professionals intersects with individuals, families, and communities. In the case of faith communities, members tend to preserve the particularity of their stories. One could argue, however, that that the ability to build networks outside of community is a valuable skill for pre-professional students. Learning to listen to the stories of these communities is an essential skill in this interaction. Faith-based initiatives have networked with the government and agencies to provide social services to neighborhoods and communities. Others have established financial and contractual relationships with other communities to rent their space. However, the formation of true community that enables mutuality might require new ways of interacting by dominant, affluent, faith communities in their relationships with less privileged

33. Fisher, "Narration, Reason, and Community," 310.
34. Ibid., 314.

groups. A willingness to listen to the stories of other communities can provide an empathic engagement to be together in community.[35]

INTERCONNECTEDNESS

Educator Mary Elizabeth Moore describes two forms of relationality. The first is the relationality of humans with the rest of the earth, where humans and all creatures deserve respect. The second is relationality across time, from generation to generation.[36] Larry Rasmussen describes the necessity of providing havens for people who seek to act morally and to create moral communities. He describes four roles of the church as a servant community of moral life, including: (1) being an inclusive community of ecumenical, egalitarian membership; (2) experimenting creatively with practices to support a new humanity in the world of interdependent strangers; (3) creating a haven or "way-station," and (4) acting as moral critic.[37]

Although empathic communities inside and outside of professional education might seem like an unattainable ideal, there is evidence of such community building around the world. One historical example is the community of Geel, Belgium, that has cared for those with mental illness in inclusive ways. Enabling the arts and creativity to transcend difference and build community is part of many local efforts that involve public art and empathy. Organizations such as Tamarack Institute for Community Engagement in Waterloo, Ontario, mobilize communities across Canada to work for common purposes, such as poverty reduction and capacity building. Examples of faith-based outreach or collaborations between faith-based agencies and the government provide situations where community goals can overcome difference.[38] Other networks include those working for aboriginal healing programs, such as Healing the Sacred and Community Healing Network, which works with African-American communities.

35. I am grateful to Rev. Michael Blair for discussions on this point.
36. Moore, *Ministering with the Earth*, 52–53.
37. Rasmussen, *Moral Fragments*.
38. Perkins, *Beyond Charity*.

COMMUNITY RESILIENCE

Prerequisites for community resilience, according to a report released by the Fetzer Foundation, are the notions of place, safety, and voice. The need for place may be described from the struggles of those who are physically displaced or those who feel lost inside. Place may also involve those who seek a sense of purpose. Safety refers to the search to find a way home and to feel at home in the world in spite of the violence that surrounds people and makes them feel insecure. The third feature is the sense of having a voice, where individuals are included in conversation and are close enough to other individuals to be heard. Community allows for the speaking and hearing of individuals in order that connections can be made. Resilience refers to the ability to survive extreme conditions "yet retain the capacity to find a way back to expressing the defining quality of *being* and the essence of *purpose*." [39] Resilience in human communities describes the capacity to forge solidarity and to meet challenges creatively, as well as "bouncing back" from adversity.

Educator Mary Gordon has piloted a school movement called "Roots of Empathy." She believes that we are born with the capacity for empathy, which grows as a child develops a sense of self. The stages in the development of empathy are: awareness of self, understanding of the emotions, ability to attribute emotions to others, and taking the perspective of the other. All of these skills are steps in developing a moral sense and a capacity for social behavior.[40] In the classroom where Gordon's program takes place, empathy is part of an atmosphere that stresses relationship, connection, and respect. By observing a baby that is brought into the classroom, the affective side of children's development is supported. Her method builds on the value of social inclusion wherein everyone has a voice. Gordon defines emotional literacy as the "ability to recognize, understand, cope with and express our emotions in appropriate ways."[41] She argues that when empathy is added to emotional literacy, we secure the basis for morally responsible behavior.

Involving professionals in the community has a number of benefits. Philosopher Charles Taylor notes that recent Western thinking detaches humans from their social environments and focuses instead on their in-

39. Pew-Fetzer, *Community Resilience*, 24.

40. Gordon, *Roots of Empathy*, 36.

41. Ibid., 117.

ternal environments and their desire to remake themselves. Community, however, is an important framework for the teaching and expression of empathy. Community is also essential to the notion of bearing witness to suffering in order that healing may occur.[42]

COMMUNITIES OF PRACTICE

Etienne Wenger defines communities of practice as groups of people who share a passion or concern for something they do and learn to do it better through regular interaction. Not all communities, in his definition, are communities of practice. In order to qualify as a community of practice, there must be a shared domain of interest or competence that distinguishes members from others. In pursuing this shared domain, members share information.

Members of communities of practice are practitioners who share information about their common practice, whether it is nursing or pastoral care. These conversations become shared repertoire for their practice. The awareness of communities of practice helps one to recognize how knowledge is managed in organizations and outside of formal structures. Educational applications of this concept of communities of practice raises questions of grounding learning in communities, namely, how to connect student experience to actual practice in communities outside of school and how to serve lifelong learning needs of students beyond graduation. In Wenger's model, learning happens outside the classroom and is situated in the world.[43]

According to Gregory Heath, the model of teaching and learning to be enlisted here is much more of doing, sharing, and practicing than of mentally possessing. Acquiring knowledge means entering into a community, whether a community of knowledge or a community of practice; indeed, it is an act of coming to be in a group and as a result locating one's understanding as part of that group. He writes that it is "the capacity to join different communities of practice with their different imaginings that provides the capacity to constitute at any particular moment our being in the world."[44]

42. Taylor, *Ethics of Authenticity*, 181.

43. Wenger, *Communities of Practice*.

44. Heath, "Exploring the Imagination," 115–23.

Although professional education views itself as part of the university or organization with which it is affiliated, there are important aspects of networking with the community that enhance the empathic connections between professionals and communities. Professional schools may encourage the involvement of students in a community of practice that may extend beyond the walls of the classroom, the college, or the students' professional training in the pursuit of a common world.

Helping students to make connections with the world in which they will eventually live and work is an important part of curriculum and professional formation. Hospitality and mutuality create a common space to share suffering, to bear witness to its reality, and to search for effective responses. In the process, the creativity and imagination of all the members will be engaged, creating new stories out of shared memories and innovative rituals that encompass the past and future.

QUESTIONS FOR FURTHER DISCUSSION

1. Define a community and provide an example.

2. Describe places where people can share a common world.

3. What types of stories are told in the communities to which you belong?

4. Have you experienced being rooted in a community? What were the things that made you feel that way?

5. Describe an incident in your education that either made you feel rooted or uprooted.

6. What kinds of things could be done in your educational or work setting to create a feeling of rootedness?

7. Do you participate in any virtual communities, such as social networking sites? How does this experience of community compare to community where there is face-to-face interaction?

8. Have you been mentored by anyone, or have you served as a mentor to someone else? What qualities does a good mentor exhibit?

9. In your workplace or school, identify two or three ways that the design of the space affects your work or how you interact with others.

10. Describe a situation in which hospitality was extended to you. How did it make you feel? How have you extended hospitality to others?

Conclusion

COMPASSION FATIGUE, EMPATHIC OVERLOAD, job stress, and burnout are frequent complaints among those in the helping professions. Although empathy can motivate one to choose a helping profession, excessive empathic engagement can also result in overload and emotional exhaustion. Those who feel overwhelmed by empathy may choose to protect themselves from potential overload by avoiding certain types of clients or by detaching from them. Others may be technically proficient but have a difficult time relating in an empathic way to a client. Sensing this distance, clients might be reluctant to share their thoughts and feelings with the practitioner. Both professional education and professional practice can have devastating effects on one's empathy, and there are few resources or mentors to whom one can honestly admit such loss.

Empathy, as a cognitive and affective skill, can be managed and learned. When empathy was previously thought to be a personality trait, many found that in the course of their professional work their personality had changed and the source of empathy seemed to run dry. Indeed, the seasons of a professional's career may include times when caring is limited to technical competence and empathy is not available. Even though empathy would thus seem to drain and exhaust a professional, when empathy is effectively managed, it can also provide a source of renewal to the practitioner.

Empathic connection requires the professional to confront his or her own suffering. Reflection and self-awareness help one to process and work through the areas in one's own life that can cause pain. It is sometimes through one's own pain that listening and empathic skills are honed. One would never choose to experience suffering for this purpose, but personal experiences of suffering can help develop aspects of empathy that energize, rather than deplete, a professional career.

Spiritual self-care is a necessity for those who confront the suffering and brokenness of the world with skills to mend bodies, spirits, or minds. Although much of our culture isolates us from some of the worst suffering, those who choose to work in helping professions find there is little buffer. Over the course of a career, regarding suffering may require a practitioner to observe some of the most painful things that one can witness. Clients who respond with anger and hatred to being helped; clients who have been restored only to self-destruct; clients whose lives are out of control and who injure vulnerable others—these are the burdens a professional must confront.

Professional schools should take responsibility for teaching students how to manage their empathic capacities, how to restore them when they are depleted, and how to practice self-care that will last through their professional lives. Space must be provided for students to honestly share and reflect on their confrontations with the brokenness of life. Such reflection is a spiritual task since it deals with questions of ultimate meaning.

Reflection, journaling, meditation practices, prayer, yoga, and art can all help to put students in touch with their own embodied response to the suffering they see and the suffering they absorb into their own bodies. Creativity can also provide innovative responses to the way things have always been done. Many change agents have regarded suffering and fought to bring about change. The ability to respond in new ways must be nurtured in professional students as well as in practicing professionals. The complexity of work environments and the rate of change require this flexibility of thinking. Thus, regarding suffering is the first task leading to empathy. The second part involves bearing witness to suffering. An affective response must be combined with cognitive skills for critical thinking, reflection, and action.

Many aspects of professional life and professional relationships provide common challenges. Students could benefit from interprofessional discussion groups or courses dealing with issues related to self-care, empathy, and bearing witness. If professionals continue to be trained in isolation from the community that they will serve or the staff with whom they will eventually work, it is unlikely that the professional boundaries that are part of the specialization that has defined the history of each profession can be overcome. There are times when an interdisciplinary or collaborative approach to suffering is needed, and such skills are better learned early in one's career. The Carnegie Foundation is currently exploring the ways that nurses and doctors could be educated interprofessionally. Students from theological schools occasionally share the classroom with health-profession students, and the interchange of perspectives is enriching. Discussions of spiritual issues tend to be restricted to courses on death and dying, but there is a greater role for spirituality in professional life, including spiritual self-care as well as ethical and moral reasoning.

Competitive values and individual success are encouraged by all the stages of professional education, from admissions to graduation. True collaboration must begin with faculty who find ways to build mutuality and cooperation in the learning culture. In addition, in order to be able to contribute to communities of practice, students must have real and prolonged contact with the communities they will serve so that their learning is both situated and applied. Students may prefer hospital placements instead of community centers, and they may cling to suburban internships rather than deal with a foreign urban or rural landscape. Mentors and field supervisors can continue to push students to encounter difference and to develop empathic skills in the process. Outcomes-based assessments have become the norm for all levels of education. The question remains how deeply such assessments affect the teaching or the learning done in classrooms. Acknowledging the different starting points of students and the very different paths each student takes to learning and formation provides a more holistic look at the curriculum. In addition, learning emphasizes and evaluates cognitive skills and markers; however, empathic abilities are more challenging to quantify and identify, and changes in those abilities as a result of the educational experience are more challenging to assess. As long as empathy is misunderstood as "niceness," the importance of empathy in the practitioner's portfolio will be underestimated. When empathy is associated with authenticity, justice, cultural competence, spirituality, authenticity, reciprocity, imagination, and creativity, one realizes that these are the skills that practitioners will need to deal with complex systems.

Practitioners do not work in an isolated setting. Relational skills that help students navigate complexity, chaos, organizations, communities, and coworkers require high levels of emotional intelligence and empathy. An understanding of the positive aspects of power, the nature of conflict, and the working of systems should be part of the practitioner's portfolio.

Is there a source of regeneration in the health-care or helping relationship that can help restore professionals or prevent burnout? Traditionally, the helper has provided care in a one-way direction. However, an empathic exchange can also acknowledge and affirm the practitioner in ways that have yet to be studied. Buber's I-thou relationship and Levinas's understanding of relationality as part of human existence suggest that in the mystery of mutual care, something transcends the individual transaction. Such regeneration can be relegated to the realm of mystery or may be described as grace. Mystery and grace may not fit the categories of scientific research, yet that does not render them invalid as categories of knowledge and experience.

When one responds to the needs of the world as an individual, the problems are simply overwhelming. If, however, students are taught to engage in communities of practice, these overwhelming problems can be addressed in creative and collaborative ways. Professional students who seek to address the larger social issues behind education and health care need mentoring to move beyond liberal guilt and the associated empathic overload. Effectively bearing witness requires a high degree of self-awareness, as well as sensitivity to the other. Humility is a key ability in learning to experience "as if" while not appropriating the experience or assuming to know better what the other is experiencing. The recognition of limits is a radical act in a modern and postmodern world—yet there are human limits to what one can understand, change, or do. Professional expertise does not provide limitless powers or abilities. The illusion of infallible practitioners has created a culture that refuses to admit mistakes.

Reflection and engagement provide a rhythm to professional life that allows for both breath and spirit. Attaining that balance is one of the most essential learning tasks for the building of empathic communities. Making room for the spirit also creates space for both grace and mystery—components that generate empathy and respect for both the earth and its inhabitants.

Making room for these values in education is the responsibility of educators and administrators and require a care for the professionals as well as the patients that is not governed by norms of overwork and over-engagement. As Dr. Nancy Angoff, Associate Dean of Student Affairs at Yale School of Medicine, eloquently notes with respect to medical education, "We ought to model and commend compassion and react to the deep feelings of our students in the same way we would teach them to react to the deep feelings of their patients—thoughtfully, respectfully, and honestly."[1] Recognitions of the affective and cognitive dimensions of empathy as well as the potential for re-creation in its application to professional life will contribute to the longevity and career satisfaction of professionals and the satisfaction of clients. Such a goal is a worthy challenge for the education of professionals as they learn to build empathic communities that work for justice.

1. Angoff, "Crying in the Curriculum," 1018.

Bibliography

Aldridge, David. *Spirituality, Healing and Medicine*. London: Jessica Kingsley, 2000.

Alma, Hans A. "Self-Development as a Spiritual Process: The Role of Empathy and Imagination in Finding Spiritual Orientation." *Pastoral Psychology* 57 (2008) 59–63.

Anderson, Herbert, and Edward Foley. *Mighty Stories, Dangerous Rituals: Weaving Together the Human and the Divine*. San Francisco: Jossey Bass, 2001.

Andre, Judith, Jake Foglio, and Howard Brody. "Moral Growth, Spirituality, and Activisim." In *Educating for Professionalism*, edited by Delise Wear and Janet Bickel, 80–94. Iowa City: University of Iowa Press, 2000.

Angoff, Nancy. "Crying in the Curriculum." *American Medical Association* 286 (2001) 1017–18.

Arendt, Hannah. *Between Past and Future*. New York: Penguin, 1977.

Atkins, S., and K. Murphy. "Reflection: A Review of the Literature." *Journal of Advanced Nursing* 18 (1993) 1188–92.

Baldwin, DeWitt. "Some Philosophical and Psychological Contributions to the Use of Self in Therapy." In *The Use of Self in Therapy*, 2nd ed., edited by Michele Baldwin, 39–60. New York: Haworth Press, 2000.

Baldwin, Michele, ed. *The Use of Self in Therapy*. 2nd ed. New York: Haworth Press, 2000.

Balint, J., and W. Shelton. "Regaining the Initiative: Forging a New Model of the Patient-Physician Relationship." *Journal of the American Medical Association* 275 (1999) 887–91.

Barker, Gary. *Adolescents, Social Support and Help-Seeking Behaviour*. Geneva: WHO, 2007.

Batson, C. D. "Prosocial Motivation: Is It Ever Truly Altruistic?" *Advances in Experimental Social Psychology* 20 (1987) 65–122.

Bauby, Jean-Dominque. *The Diving Bell and the Butterfly*. New York: Random House, 1998.

Benner, Patricia. *From Novice to Expert: Excellence and Power in Clinical Nursing Practice*. Menlo Park, CA: Addison-Wesley, 1984.

Benner, Patricia, Molly Sutphen, Victoria Leonard, and Lisa Day. *Educating Nurses: A Call for Radical Transformation*. San Francisco: Jossey-Bass, 2009.

Bennett, Michael, ed. *The Empathic Healer*. New York: Academic Press, 2001.

Bhui, K. "The Language of Compliance: Health Policy and Clinical Practice for the Severely Mentally Ill." *International Journal of Social Psychiatry* 43 (1997) 157–63.

Blackford, Jeanine. "Cultural Frameworks of Nursing Practice: Exposing an Exclusionary Healthcare Culture." *Nursing Inquiry* 10 (2003) 236–44.

Block, Peter. *Community: The Structure of Belonging*. San Francisco: Berrett-Kohler, 2008.

Blum, Lawrence. "Value Underpinnings of Antiracist and Multicultural Education." In *Systems of Education: Theories, Policies and Implicit Values*, edited by Mal Leicester, 4–14. London: Falmer, 2000.

Boler, M., and M. Zembylas. "Discomforting Truths: The Emotional Terrain of Understanding Differences." In *Pedagogies of Difference: Rethinking Education for Social Justice*, edited by P. Trifonas. New York: Routledge, 2003.

Bowker, John. *Problems of Suffering in Religions of the World*. Cambridge: Cambridge University Press, 1970.

Bozarth, Jerold D. "Empathy from the Framework of Client-Centered Theory and the Rogerian Hypothesis." In *Empathy Reconsidered: New Directions in Psychotherapy*, edited by Arthur Bohart and L. Greenberg. Washington, DC: American Psychological Association, 1997.

Brookfield, Stephen. *Becoming a Critically Reflective Teacher*. San Francisco: Jossey-Bass, 1995.

———. *Developing Critical Thinkers*. San Francisco: Jossey-Bass, 1987.

Brown, Brené. *I Thought It Was Just Me: Women Reclaiming Power and Courage in a Culture of Shame*. New York: Gotham, 2007.

Brueggeman, Walter. *Peace*. St. Louis: Chalice, 2001.

Brus, H., M. Van de Laar, E. Taal, J. Rasker, and O. Wiegman. "Compliance in Rheumatoid Arthritis and the Role of Formal Patient Education." *Seminars in Arthritis and Rheumatism* 26 (1997) 702–10.

Buber, Martin. *I and Thou*. Translated by Walter Kaufman. New York: Charles Scribner's Sons, 1970.

Burkhart, Patricia, and Mary Kay Rayens. "Self Concept and Health Locus of Control: Factors Related to Children's Adherence to Recommended Asthma Regimen." *Pediatric Nursing* 31 (2005) 404–10.

Candib, Lucy M. "Reconsidering Power in the Clinical Relationship." In *The Empathic Practitioner*, edited by Ellen Singer More and Maureen A. Milligan, 135–56. New Brunswick, NJ: Rutgers University Press, 1994.

Cassell, Eric J. *The Nature of Suffering and the Goals of Medicine*. New York: Oxford University Press, 1991.

Cates, Diana Fritz. *Choosing to Feel: Virtue, Friendship, and Compassion for Friends*. Notre Dame: University of Notre Dame Press, 1997.

Chapman, K. R., S. Cluel, and L. Fabri. "Improving Patient Compliance with Asthma Therapy." *Respiratory Medicine* 94 (2000) 2–9.

Charon, Rita. *Narrative Medicine*. New York: Oxford, 2006.

———. *Stories Matter: The Role of Narrative in Medical Ethics*. New York: Routledge, 2002.

Chen, Pauline W. "Do You Have the Right Stuff to Be a Doctor?" *New York Times*, 15 January 2010.

Cherry, Conrad. *Hurrying toward Zion: Universities, Divinity Schools, and American Protestantism*. Bloomington: Indiana University Press, 1995.

Chickering, Arthur W., Jon C. Dalton, and Liesa Stamm. *Encouraging Authenticity and Spirituality in Higher Education*. San Francisco: John Wiley & Sons, 2006.

Chinnery, Ann, and Heesoon Bai. "Altering Conceptions of Subjectivity." In *Systems of Education: Theories, Policies and Implicit Values*, 86–96. London: Falmer, 2000.

Chubbuck, Sharon M., and Michalinos Zembylas. "The Emotional Ambivalence of Socially Just Teaching: A Case Study of a Novice Urban Schoolteacher." *American Educational Research Journal* 45 (2008) 274–318.

Code, Lorraine. "'I Know Just How You Feel': Empathy and the Problem of Epistemic Authority." In *The Empathic Practitioner*, edited by Ellen Singer More and Maureen A. Milligan, 77–97. New Brunswick, NJ: Rutgers University Press, 1994.

———. *What Can She Know? Feminist Theory and the Construction of Knowledge.* Ithaca: Cornell University Press, 1991.

Coles, Robert. *Dorothy Day: A Radical Devotion.* Reading, MA: Perseus, 1987.

Comer, James P. *Beyond Black and White.* New York: Quadrangle Books, 1972.

———. *Maggie's American Dream: The Life and Times of an American Black Family.* New York: Plume, 1989.

———. *What I Learned in School: Reflections on Race, Child Development, and School Reform.* San Francisco: Jossey-Bass, 2009.

Connelly, Julia E. "The Empathic Practitioner: Empathy, Gender, and Medicine." In *The Empathic Practitioner*, edited by Ellen Singer More and Maureen A. Milligan, 171–88. New Brunswick, NJ: Rutgers University Press, 1994.

Coutts, Mary Carrington. "Teaching Ethics in the Health Care Setting Part I: Survey of the Literature." *Kennedy Institute of Ethics Journal* 1 (1991) 171–85.

Craig, Robert. *Philosophical and Educational Foundations in a Multicultural Society.* Waterbury, CT: Emancipation Press, 1999.

Curry-Stevens, Ann. "New Forms of Transformative Education: Pedagogy for the Privileged." *Journal of Transformative Education* 5 (2007) 33–58.

Daloz Parks, Sharon. *Big Questions, Worthy Dreams: Mentoring Young Adults in Their Search for Meaning, Purpose, and Faith.* San Francisco: Jossey-Bass, 2000.

Dalton, Jon C. "Integrating Spirit and Community in Higher Education." In *Encouraging Authenticity and Higher Education*, edited by Arthur W. Chickering, Jon C. Dalton and Liesa Stamm, 165–86. San Francisco: Jossey-Bass, 2006.

Das, Veena, Arthur Kleinman, Margaret Lock, Mamphala Ramphele, and Pamela Reynolds, eds. *Remaking a World: Violence, Social Suffering, and Recovery.* Berkeley: University of California Press, 2001.

Davis, Mark. *Empathy: A Social Psychological Approach.* Boulder, CO: Westview, 1996.

Day, Dorothy. *Loaves and Fishes.* Maryknoll, NY: Orbis, 1963.

———. *The Long Loneliness: An Autobiography.* New York: Harper and Row, 1952.

Dayringer, Richard. *The Heart of Pastoral Counseling.* Grand Rapids, MI: Ministry Resources Library, 1989.

Deloughery, Grace. *Issues and Trends in Nursing.* 2nd ed. St. Louis: Mosby, 1997.

Di Matteo, M. R., Kelly Haskard, and Summer Williams. "Health Beliefs, Disease Severity, and Patient Adherence." *Medical Care* 45 (2007) 521–28.

Doornbos, Mary Molewyk, Ruth E. Groenhout, and Kendra Hotz. *Transforming Care: A Christian Vision of Nursing Practice.* Grand Rapids, MI: Eerdmans, 2005.

Doyle, Clar, and Amarjit Singh. *Reading and Teaching Henry Giroux.* New York: Peter Lang, 2006.

Easter, Anna. "Construct Analysis of Four Modes of Being Present." *Journal of Holistic Nursing* 18 (2000) 362–77.

Eisenthal, S., R. Emery, A. Lazare, and H. Udin. "'Adherence' and the Negotiated Approach to Parenthood." *Archives of General Psychiatry* 36 (1979) 393–98.

English, L. M., Tara J. Fenwick, and Jim Parsons. *Spirituality of Adult Education and Training.* Malabar, FL: Krieger, 2003.

Everding, H. Edward, and Lucinda Huffaker. "Educating Adults for Empathy: Implications of Cognitive Role-Taking and Identity Formation." *Religious Education* 93 (1998) 413–30.

Farley, Margaret. *Compassionate Respect*. Mahwah, NJ: Paulist Press, 2002.

Farmer, Paul. *Pathologies of Power: Health, Human Rights, and the New War on the Poor*. Berkeley: University of California Press, 2005.

Farrell, Marian, and Mary E. Muscari. "Empathy." In *Developing Professional Behaviors*, edited by Jack Kasar and E. Nelson Clark, 65–73. Thorofare, NJ: Slack, 2000.

Fenichel, Otto. *The Psychoanalytic Theory of Neurosis*. New York: W. W. Norton and Company, 1945.

Feshbach, Norma Deitch. "Empathy: The Formative Years—Implications for Clinical Practice." In *Empathy Reconsidered: New Directions in Psychotherapy*, edited by Arthur Bohart and L. Greenberg, 33–59. Washington, D.C.: American Psychological Association, 1997.

Fisher, Walter R. "Narration, Reason, and Community." In *Memory, Identity, Community: The Idea of Narrative in the Human Sciences*, edited by Lewis P. Hinchman and Sanda K. Hinchman, 307–27. Albany: State University of New York Press, 1997.

Fortin, Auguste, and Katherine Gergen Barnett. "Medical School Curricula in Spirituality and Medicine." *JAMA* 291 (2004) 2883.

Foster, Charles R., Lisa E. Dahill, Lawrence A. Golemon, and Barbara Wang, eds. *Educating Clergy: Teaching Practices and Pastoral Imagination*. Stanford, CA: Jossey-Bass, 2006.

Fowler, James. *Stages of Faith*. San Francisco: Harper and Row, 1981.

Frank, Arthur. *The Wounded Storyteller*. Chicago: University of Chicago Press, 1995.

Freidson, Eliot. *Professionalism: The Third Logic*. Cambridge: Polity, 2001.

Freire, Paulo. *Pedagogy of the Oppressed*. Translated by M. Berman Ramos. New York: Herder and Herder, 1970.

Gallese, Vittorio. "Intentional Attunement: Mirror Neurons and the Neural Underpinnings of Interpersonal Relations." *Journal of the American Psychoanalytic Association* 55 (2007) 131–75.

Gidney, William, and W. P. J. Millar. *Professional Gentlemen: The Professions in Nineteenth-Century Ontario*. Toronto: University of Toronto Press, 1994.

Giroux, Henry. "Cultural Studies, Public Pedagogy, and the Responsibility of Intellectuals." *Communication and Critical/Cultural Studies* 1 (2004) 59–79.

———. "The War against Children and the Shredding of the Social Contract." In *Communities of Difference*, edited by Peter P. Trifonas, 3–26. New York: Palgrave MacMillan, 2005.

Gochman, David S. *Health Behavior: Emerging New Perspectives*. New York: Plenum, 1998.

Goleman, Daniel. *Social Intelligence*. New York: Bantam, 2006.

Goodman, Diane. *Promoting Diversity and Social Justice: Educating People from Privileged Groups*. Thousand Oaks, CA: Sage Publications, 2001.

Gordon, Mary. *Roots of Empathy*. Toronto: Thomas Allen, 2005.

Greene, Maxine. *Releasing the Imagination*. San Francisco: Jossey-Bass, 1995.

Haberman, Mel. "Suffering and Survivorship." In *Suffering*, edited by Betty Rolling Ferrell, 121–42. Sudbury, MA: Jones and Bartlett, 1996.

Hall, Douglas John. *God and Human Suffering*. Minneapolis: Augsburg, 1986.

Halpern, Jodi. *From Detached Concern to Empathy: Humanizing Medical Practice*. New York: Oxford, 2001.

Hardee, James T. "An Overview of Empathy." *Permanente Journal* 7 (2003). Online: http://xnet.kp.org/permanentejournal/fall03/cpc.html.

Haynes, B. R., W. R. Taylor, and D. L. Sackett. *Compliance in Health Care*. Baltimore, MD: Johns Hopkins Press, 1979.

Heath, Gregory. "Exploring the Imagination to Establish Frameworks for Learning." *Studies in Philosophical Education* 27 (2008) 115–23.

Heemskerk, Margaretha. *Suffering in Mutazilite Theology*. Leiden: E. J. Brill, 2000.

Herman, Judith Lewis. *Trauma and Recovery*. New York: Basic, 1997.

Hertogh, C. M. "The Loss of a Common Shared World: Ethical Problems in Palliative Care for People with Advanced Dementia." *Journal of Gerontology and Geriatrics [Tijdschr Gerontol Geriatr]* 39 (2008) 265–72.

Hess, D. J. "The Ethics of Compliance: A Dialectic." *Advance in Nursing Science* 19 (1996) 18–27.

Hinchman, Lewis P., and Sandra K. Hinchman, eds. *Memory, Idenity, Community: The Idea of Narrative in the Human Sciences*. Albany: State University of New York Press, 1997.

Hine, Darlene Clark. *Black Women in White: Racial Conflict and Cooperation in the Nursing Profession, 1890–1950*. Bloomington: Indiana University Press, 1989.

Hoffman, Martin L. *Empathy and Moral Development*. Cambridge: Cambridge University Press, 2000.

Hojat, Mohammadreza. *Empathy in Patient Care*. New York: Springer, 2007.

Holman, Susan R. *God Knows There's Need: Christian Responses to Poverty*. Oxford: Oxford University Press, 2009.

Holmes, Dave and D. Gastaldo. "Rhizomatic Thought in Nursing: An Alternative Path for the Development of the Discipline." *Nursing Philosophy* 5 (2004): 258–67.

hooks, bell. *Where We Stand: Class Matters*. New York: Routledge, 2000.

Huffaker, Lucinda Stark. *Creative Dwelling: Empathy and Clarity in God and Self*. Atlanta, GA: Scholars Press, 1998.

Institute of Medicine. *In the Nation's Compelling Interest*. Washington, D.C., 2004.

Jacobs, L. "Personal Knowing in Cancer Nursing." *Nursing Forum* 33 (1998) 23–28.

Jones, Serene. *Trauma and Grace: Theology in a Ruptured World*. Louisville, KY: Westminster John Knox, 2009.

Jordan, Judith, ed. *Women's Growth in Diversity: More Writings from the Stone Center*. New York: Guilford, 1997.

Kahn, David L., and Richard Steeves. "An Understanding of Suffering Grounded in Clinical Practice and Research." In *Suffering*, edited by Betty Rolling Ferrell, 3–28. Sudbury, MA: Jones and Bartlett, 1996.

Kanpol, Barry, and Peter McLaren. "Multiculturalism and Empathy: A Border Pegagogy of Solidarity." In *Critical Multiculturalism: Uncommon Voices in a Common Struggle*, edited by Barry Kanpol and Peter McLaren, 177–95. Westport, CT: Bergin & Garvey, 1995.

Katz, J. *The Silent World of Doctor and Patient*. New York: Free Press, 1984.

Kazanowski, Mary, Kathleen Perrin, Mertie Potter, and Caryn Sheehan. "The Silence of Suffering." *Journal of Holistic Nursing* 25 (2007) 195–203.

Keith, Heather. "Transforming Ren: The De of George Herbert Mead's Social Self." *Journal of Chinese Philosophy* 36 (2009) 69–84.

Kelly, Thomas R. *A Testament of Devotion*. San Francisco: Harper & Bros., 1992.

Kessler, Shelley. *The Teaching Presence*. Vol. 4. Holistic Education Review (1991) 1–15. Online: http://passageworks.org/wp-content/uploads/file/UnpublishedTeaching Presence.pdf.

Kinnear, Mary. *In Subordination: Professional Women, 1870–1970*. Montreal: McGill-Queen's University Press, 1995.

Klass, Perri. "The Empathic Practitioner." In *The Empathic Practitioner*, edited by Ellen Singer More and Maureen A. Milligan, 157–70. New Brunswick, NJ: Rutgers University Press, 1994.

Kleinman, Arthur. *The Illness Narrative: Suffering, Healing and the Human Condition*. New York: Basic, 1988.

———. *Writing at the Margin: Discourse between Anthropology and Medicine*. Berkeley: University of California Press, 1995.

Kleinman, Arthur, Veena Das, and Margaret Lock. *Social Suffering*. Berkeley: University of California Press, 1997.

Kohn, Alfie. *Beyond Discipline: From Compliance to Community*. Alexandria, VA: ASCD, 2006.

Kohut, H. *The Analysis of the Self*. New York: International Universities Press, 1971.

Koslowski, P. *The Origins and Overcoming of Evil and Suffering in the World Religions*. New York: Springer, 2001.

Kubler-Ross, Elizabeth. *On Death and Dying*. New York: MacMillan, 1969.

Kuhse, Helga. *Caring: Nurses, Women and Ethics*. Oxford: Blackwell, 1997.

Lampert, Khen. *Traditions of Compassion: From Religious Duty to Social Activism*. Hampshire: Palgrave MacMillan, 2005.

Leggo, Carl. "The Letter of the Law / the Silence of Letters: Poetic Ruminations on Love and School." In *Communities of Difference*, edited by Peter P. Trifonas, 107–26. New York: Palgrave MacMillan, 2005.

Lerner, Barron H. "From Careless Consumptives to Recalcitrant Patients: The Historical Construction of Compliance." *Social Science and Medicine* 45 (1998) 1423–31.

Levinson, Natasha. "The Paradox of Natality: Teaching in the Midst of Belatedness." In *Hannah Arendt and Education: Renewing Our Common World*, 11–36. Boulder, CO: Westview, 2001.

Lock, Margaret. "Medical Knowledge and Body Politics." In *Exotic No More: Anthropology on the Front Lines*, edited by Jeremy MacClancy. Chicago: University of Chicago Press, 2002.

Luft, F. C., C. D. Morris, and M. H. Weinberger. "Compliance to a Low-Salt Diet." *American Journal of Clinical Nutrition* 64 (1997) 698S–703S.

Lutfey, Karen E., and William J. Wishner. "Beyond 'Compliance' Is 'Adherence': Improving the Prospect of Diabetes Care." *Diabetes Care* 22 (1999) 635–39.

MacIssac, David S. "Empathy: Heinz Kohut's Contribution." In *Empathy Reconsidered: New Directions in Pscyhotherapy*, edited by Arthur Bohart and L. Greenberg, 245–64. Washington, D.C.: American Psychological Association, 1997.

Macy, Joanna. *Coming Back to Life: Practices to Reconnect Our Lives, Our World*. Gabriola Island, BC: New Society, 1998.

———. *Widening Circles*. Gabriola Island, BC: New Society, 2000.

Maich, Nancy Matthew. "'Becoming' through Reflection and Professional Portfolios: The Voice of Growth in Nurses." *Reflective Practice* 1 (2000) 309–24.

Marck, Patricia. "Therapeutic Reciprocity: A Caring Phenomenon." *Advanced Nursing Science* 13 (1990) 49–59.

May, Rollo. *The Courage to Create*. New York: W. W. Norton and Co., 1975.

McDougall, William. *Introduction to Social Psychology*. London: Metheun and Co., 1908.

McNeill, William. *Plagues and Peoples*. Garden City, NY: Anchor, 1998.

Mead, George Herbert. *Mind, Self, and Society: From the Standpoint of a Social Behaviorist*. Chicago: University of Chicago Press, 1934.

Meleis, A. I. *Theoretical Nursing: Development and Progress*. New York: Lippincott, 1997.

Meyer, Elaine C., Deborah E. Sellers, David M. Browning, Kimberly McGuffie, Mildred Z. Solomon, and Robert D. Truog. "Difficult Conversations: Improving Communication Skills and Relational Abilities in Health Care." *Pediatric Critical Care Medicine* 10 (2009) 352–59.

Mezirow, Jack. *Learning as Transformation*. San Francisco: Jossey-Bass, 2000.

———. *Transformative Dimensions of Adult Learning*. San Francisco: Jossey-Bass, 1991.

Miller, J. "Learning from a Spiritual Perspective." In *Expanding the Boundaries of Transformative Learning*, edited by Edmund O'Sullivan, 95–102. New York: Palgrave, 2002.

Mitchem, Stephanie Y., and Emilie M. Townes, eds. *Faith, Health, and Healing in African American Life*. Religion, Faith, and Healing. Westport, CT: Praeger, 2008.

Modell, Arnold H. *Imagination and the Meaningful Brain*. Cambridge, MA: MIT Press, 2003.

Moore, Mary Elizabeth. *Ministering with the Earth*. St. Louis: Chalice, 1998.

Morantz-Sanchez, Regina Markell. *Sympathy and Science: Women Physicians in American Medicine*. Chapel Hill: University of North Carolina, 2000.

More, Ellen Singer, and Maureen A. Milligan, eds. *The Empathic Practitioner: Empathy, Gender, and Medicine*. New Brunswick, NJ: Rutgers University Press, 1994.

Nagata, Donna K. *Legacy of Injustice: Exploring the Cross-Generational Impact of the Japanese American Internment*. New York: Plenum Press, 1993.

Nash, Robert. *Spirituality, Ethics and Teaching*. New York: Peter Lang, 2002.

Neilson, A. R., and D. K. Whynes. "Determinants of Persistent Compliance with Screening for Colorectal Cancer." *Social Science Medicine* 41 (1995) 365–74.

Nouwen, Henri. *Adam: God's Beloved*. Maryknoll, NY: Orbis, 1997.

O'Connell, Maureen H. *Compassion: Loving Our Neighbor in an Age of Globalization*. Maryknoll, NY: Orbis, 2009.

Orbinski, James. *An Imperfect Offering*. Toronto: Anchor Canada, 2008.

Palmer, Parker. *The Active Life*. San Francisco: Jossey-Bass, 1990.

———. *Let Your Life Speak: Listening for the Voice of Vocation*. San Francisco: Jossey-Bass, 2000.

———. *To Know as We Are Known: Education as a Spiritual Journey*. San Francisco: HarperSan Francisco, 1993.

Park, Crystal, Bennett Moehl, Juliane Fenster, D. P. Suresh, and Debbie Bliss. "Religiousness and Treatment Adherence in Congestive Heart Failure Patients." *Journal of Religion, Spirituality, and Aging* 20 (2008) 249–66.

Parsons, Sharon, P. Cruise, W. Davenport, and Vanessa Jones. "Religious Beliefs, Practices, and Treatment Adherence among Individuals with HIV in the Southern United States." *AIDS Patient Care* 20 (2006) 97–111.

Peck, M. Scott. *The Different Drum*. New York: Simon and Schuster, 1987.

Perkins, John M. *Beyond Charity: The Call to Christian Community Development*. Grand Rapids, MI: Baker, 1993.

Pew-Fetzer. *Community Resilience: A Cross-Cultural Study.* Washington, D.C.: Woodrow Wilson International Center for Scholars, 2009.

Puchalski, Christine, Betty Ferrell, Rose Virani, Shirley Otis-Green, Pamela Baird, Janet Bull, and Harvey Chochinov. "Improving the Quality of Spiritual Care as a Dimension of Palliative Care: The Report of the Consensus Conference." *Journal of Palliative Medicine* 12 (2009) 885–904.

Purpel, David. *The Moral and Spiritual Crisis in Education.* New York: Bergin and Garvey, 1989.

Rasmussen, Larry. *Moral Fragments and Moral Community: A Proposal for Church in Society.* Minneapolis: Fortress, 1993.

Reisinger, Ernest. "The New Testament Meaning of 'Witness.'" *Founders Journal* 5 (1991). Online: http://www.founders.org/journal/fj05/contents.html.

Reynolds, Thomas. *Vulnerable Communion: A Theology of Disability and Hospitality.* Grand Rapids, MI: Brazos, 2008.

Richards, Ruth, ed. *Everyday Creativity and New Views of Human Nature.* Washington, DC: American Psychological Association, 2007.

Robertson, Douglas L. "Facilitating Transformative Learning: Attending to the Dynamics of the Educational Helping Relationship." *Adult Education Quarterly* 47 (1996) 41–53.

Rogers, Carl R. *Counselling and Psychotherapy.* Cambridge, MA: Riverside Press, 1942.

Rossiter, Margaret. *Women Scientists in America: Struggles and Strategies to 1940.* Baltimore: Johns Hopkins Press, 1981.

Rovira, Josep Puig. "Diversity and Universal Values in Multicultural Education." In *Systems of Education: Theories, Policies and Implicit Values,* edited by Mal Leicester, 73–81. London: Falmer, 2000.

Ruddick, Sara. "Maternal Thinking." In *Mothering. Essays in Feminist Theory,* edited by Joyce Trebilcot, 213–30. Totawa, NJ: Rowman & Allenheld, 1983.

Salovey, Peter, Marc Brackett, and John Mayer. *Emotional Intelligence: Key Readings on the Mayer and Salovey Method.* Port Chester, NY: Dude, 2004.

Salzman, C. "Medication Compliance in the Elderly." *Journal of Clinical Psychiatry* 56 (1995) 18–22.

Santacroce, Sheila, and Ya-Ling Lee. "Uncertainty, Posttraumatic Stress, and Health Behavior in Young Childhood Cancer Survivors." *Nursing Research* 55 (2006) 259–66.

Scheper-Hughes, Nancy. *Death without Weeping: The Violence of Everyday Life in Brazil.* Berkeley: University of California Press, 1992.

Schön, Donald. *The Reflective Practitioner.* New York: Basic Books, 1983.

Schutz, Aaron. "Contesting Utopianism: Hannah Arendt and the Tensions of Democratic Education." In *Hannah Arendt and Education: Renewing Our Common World,* edited by Mordechai Gordon, 93–125. Boulder, CO: Westview, 2001.

Selles, Johanna. "The Concept of Dukkha in Early Buddhism." Hamilton, ON: McMaster University, 1984.

———. "The Concept of History in Hannah Arendt." Hamilton, ON: McMaster University, 1983.

———. "The Concept of Suffering in Samkhya." Hamilton, ON: McMaster University, 1984.

———. "The Spirituality of Labour." M.Phil.F thesis, Institute for Christian Studies, 1983.

Singer, Merrill, and Hans Baer. *Introducing Medical Anthropology*. New York: Altamira Press, 2007.

Singh, Basil. "Cultural Pluralism as an Educational Ideal." In *Systems of Education: Theories, Policies and Implicit Values*, edited by Mal Leicester, 58–72. London: Falmer Press, 2000.

Smith, Robert. "Theological Perspectives." In *Suffering*, edited by Betty Rolling Ferrell, 159–72. Sudbury, MA: Jones and Bartlett, 1996.

Sobrino, Jon. *The Principle of Mercy*. Maryknoll, NY: Orbis, 1994.

Soelle, Dorothee. *Suffering*. Translated by Everett R. Kalin. Philadelphia: Fortress Press, 1975.

Sontag, Susan. *Regarding the Pain of Others*. New York: Picador, 2003.

Spelman, Elizabeth. *Fruits of Sorrow: Framing Our Attention to Suffering*. Boston: Beacon, 1997.

Spencer, Herbert. *The Principles of Psychology*. London: Williams and Norgate, 1870.

Sperry, Len. *Spirituality in Clinical Practice*. New York: Routledge, 2001.

Spink, Kathryn. *The Miracle, the Message, the Story: Jean Vanier and L'Arche*. Toronto, Ontario: Novalis, 2006.

Spiro, Howard, Mary G. McCrea, Enid Peschel, and Deborah St. James, eds. *Empathy and the Practice of Medicine*. New Haven, CT: Program for the Humanities in Medicine, 1993.

Spross, Judith A. "Coaching and Suffering: The Role of the Nurse in Helping People Face Illness." In *Suffering*, edited by Betty Rolling Ferrell, 173–208. Sudbury, MA: Jones and Bartlett, 1996.

"Standards for the Therapeutic Nurse-Client Relationship." Edited by Nurses Association of New Brunswick. Moncton, NB, 2000.

Stepien, A., and A. Baernstein. "Educating for Empathy: A Review." *Journal of General Internal Medicine* 21 (2006) 524–30.

Stotland, Ezra, Kenneth E. Matthews, Stanley Sherman, Robert O. Hansson, and Barbara Z. Richardson. *Empathy, Fantasy and Helping*. Beverly Hills, CA: Sage Publications, 1978.

Suchman, A. L. "What Makes the Patient-Doctor Relationship Therapeutic? Exploring the Connexional Dimension of Medical Care." *Annals of Internal Medicine* 108 (1998) 125–30.

Sullivan, Harry Stack. *The Interpersonal Theory of Psychiatry*. New York: W. W. Norton, 1953.

Szasz, T. S., and M. H. Hollender. "A Contribution to the Philosophy of Medicine: The Basic Models of the Doctor-Patient Relationship." *Archives of Internal Medicine* 97 (1956) 585–92.

Taylor, Charles. *The Ethics of Authenticity*. Cambridge, MA: Harvard University Press, 1992.

Thackara, John. *In the Bubble: Designing in a Complex World*. Cambridge, MA: MIT Press, 2005.

Thompson, Darren, and Paul Ciechanowski. "Attaching a New Understanding to the Patient-Physician Relationship in Family Practice." *Journal of the American Board of Family Practice* 16 (2003) 219–26.

Thorne, Sally, and Barbara Patterson. "Shifting Imagines of Chronic Illness." *Journal of Nursing Scholarship* 30 (1998) 173–78.

Thurman, Howard. *Jesus and the Disinherited*. Boston: Beacon Press, 1996.

Thurman, Howard. *With Head and Heart: The Autobiography of Howard Thurman.* San Diego: Mariner, 1981.

———. "Mysticism and Social Action." In *Lawrence Lectures on Religion and Society*, 14–35. Kensington, CA: First Unitarian Church of Berkeley, 1978.

Tisdell, Elizabeth. *Exploring Spirituality and Culture in Adult and Higher Education.* San Francisco: Jossey-Bass, 2003.

Travelbee, Joyce. *Interpersonal Aspects of Nursing.* Philadelphia: F. A. Davis, 1971.

Van Maanen, M. *Researching Lived Experiences.* London: Althouse, 1990.

Veatch, R. M., and S. Sollitto. "Medical Ethics Teaching: Report of a National Medical School Survey." *JAMA* 235 (1991) 1030–33.

Wald, Florence, and Henry Wald. Manuscript Group 1659. Yale University Manuscripts and Archives.

Wald, Florence. "Proceedings of a Conference at Yale School of Nursing: 'A Nurse's Study of Care for Dying Patients.'" Yale University Manuscripts and Archives, 1970.

Wallace, Lane. "Multicultural Critical Theory. At B-School?" *New York Times*, 10 January 2010.

Ward-Collins, D. "Noncompliant: Isn't There a Better Way to Say It?" *American Journal of Nursing* 98 (1998) 27–31.

Warner, Margaret S. "Does Empathy Cure? A Theoretical Consideration of Empathy, Processing, and Personal Narrative." In *Empathy Reconsidered: New Directions in Pscyhotherapy*, edited by Arthur Bohart and L. Greenberg, 125–40. Washington, D.C.: American Psychological Association, 1997.

Watson, Jean. *Nursing: Human Science and Human Care.* New York: National League for Nursing, 1988.

Weil, Simone. *Gravity and Grace.* London: Routledge and Kegan Paul, 1972.

———. *The Need for Roots: Prelude to a Declaration of Duties toward Mankind.* Translated by Arthur Wills. New York: G. P. Putnam's Sons, 1952.

Wenger, Etienne. *Communities of Practice: Learning, Meaning, and Identity.* Cambridge: Cambridge University Press, 1998.

Wiesel, Elie. *Night.* New York: Bantam, 1982.

Wiseman, Theresa. "A Concept Analysis of Empathy." *Journal of Advanced Nursing* 23 (1996) 1162–67.

Woodgate, R. L., and L. F. Degner. "Expectations and Beliefs about Children's Cancer Symptoms: Perspectives of Children with Cancer and Their Families." *Oncology Nursing Forum* 30 (2003) 479–91.

Wright, Stephen, and Jean Sayre Adams. *Sacred Space: Right Relations and Spirituality.* London: Churchill Livingstone, 1999.

Young, William P. *The Shack.* Newbury Park, CA: Windblown Media, 2007.

Zaltz, Freya. "Authenticity in Education: Morality, Learning, and Social Change." Paper presented at the Canadian Association for the Study of Adult Education, OISE, Toronto, 2003.

Index

www.ingramcontent.com/pod-product-compliance
Lightning Source LLC
Chambersburg PA
CBHW071100280326
41928CB00050B/2574